INTERMITTENT FASTING FOR WOMEN OVER 50

Unlock the Secrets to Burning Belly Fat, Balancing Hormones, Transforming Your Physique, and Detoxifying Your Body Using a 14-Day Meal Plan + Yummy Recipes.

SAVANNAH USHER

TABLE OF CONTENTS

<u>14-Day Meal Plan</u>

Introduction

A Welcome Message

Welcome to "Intermittent Fasting for Women Over 50," a rejuvenation, health, and vitality journey designed exclusively for the extraordinary women entering their golden years.

It is truly a pleasure to embark on this journey with you as we investigate the tremendous effects on wellbeing and the transformational potential of intermittent fasting. Designed to meet the specific requirements of women navigating the colorful tapestry of life after 50, this book is more than simply a handbook; it's a traveling companion on your journey to adopting a healthier lifestyle.

As you turn these pages, envision a roadmap designed to harness the synergy between intermittent fasting and the wisdom gained through the years. This isn't about restrictive diets or fleeting trends; it's about embracing a sustainable approach that aligns with the grace and strength inherent in every woman.

When adapted to the unique path of women over 50, intermittent fasting—often hailed for its capacity to boost metabolism and encourage cellular repair—takes on a new significance. We'll explore the complexities of this way of life in the pages that follow, comprehending its physiological subtleties and creating customized plans that flow naturally with the ups and downs of life's seasons.

Think of this book as your guide as you navigate the art of creating wholesome meals, the science of intermittent fasting, and the delight of rediscovering your identity. It's important to understand why this method is specifically tailored to improve your general vitality, energy levels, and well-being rather than just the what and how.

Discover relevant tales of women who have traveled this journey among the abundance of knowledge; learn about their victories, hardships, and the overwhelming sense of empowerment that results from adopting a way of life that prioritizes health. Both your trip and the advice found in these pages are unique.

With an open mind and a curious heart, approach this book. Examine the chapters as discussions with a buddy who is familiar with the nuances of your life, body, and goals rather than as a list of directions. We will walk through the challenges of intermittent fasting together, appreciating the uniqueness of your experience and the strength that comes from women all around the world joining you on this inspiring path.

This is an invitation, dear reader, to develop timeless wellness, appreciate the beauty that is present in every stage of life, and find a renewed sense of vigor. Together, let's set out on this adventure and embrace the potential of intermittent fasting as a beacon of hope for a thriving future.

Importance of Intermittent Fasting for Women Over 50

Women over 50 are in a unique position where their health and well-being are of utmost importance. Let me introduce you to intermittent fasting, a technique that becomes a reliable ally throughout this wonderful stage of life and has many advantages beyond the traditional dieting conventions.

The ability of intermittent fasting for women over 50 to adjust to the changing requirements of an aging body is one of its most impressive features. Hormonal balances change, our metabolism changes, and health issues become more important as we age gracefully. As a customized strategy, intermittent fasting may adapt to these shifts with a level of grace that traditional diets frequently lack.

Fundamentally, intermittent fasting is a holistic lifestyle strategy that takes advantage of the body's natural ability for regeneration rather than merely being a calorie restriction. This approach uses a controlled feeding and fasting schedule to stimulate the mechanisms involved in cellular repair. This could lead to an improvement in general well-being for women over 50, supporting longevity and helping to maintain essential body processes.

The importance of intermittent fasting in this population is further supported by a large body of research evidence. Research indicates that judicious fasting may be essential for controlling weight, a factor that is becoming more and more important for preserving health and preventing age-related issues. It benefits not only the physical aspects but also cognitive function and may lower the risk of neurodegenerative disorders.

Crucially, there is no one-size-fits-all approach to intermittent fasting for women over 50. It acknowledges the originality of every woman's journey and the particular dietary requirements and hormonal swings associated with this time of life. This flexibility enables a customized approach, guaranteeing that the fasting regimen harmonizes with an individual's tastes, lifestyle, and health objectives.

Furthermore, intermittent fasting is a welcome diversion from the frequently complicated and restrictive nature of regular diets. It encourages a better mindset and attentive eating, calling for a revitalized connection with food. This method offers women over 50 release from the constraints of traditional dietary conventions and a fun, sustainable way to nourish their bodies.

Intermittent fasting essentially acts as a wellness beacon, pointing the way toward improved health, vigor, and a more satisfying existence. It's a comprehensive embracing of wellbeing rather than only a nutritional plan, enabling women to relish this chapter's richness with dignity and fortitude.

Brief Overview of the Book

This book is a celebration of resilience, accepting change, and wisely caring for your body—it's not only about losing weight. We explore the essence of intermittent fasting via a warm and encouraging lens, dispelling its myths and revealing its significant influence on the particular requirements of women over fifty.

Learn about the intriguing interactions that occur between your body's complex hormone dance and intermittent fasting. By delving further into the physiological subtleties, we uncover how this strategy complements the normal aging process by improving cellular repair, metabolism, and vitality. Instead of offering a one-size-fits-all solution, we create a unique roadmap that honors your uniqueness while tackling the difficulties and appreciating the pleasures of the journey.

The main focus of this excursion is the delicious food. We go into the practice of enjoying nutrient-dense foods, striking a balance between macronutrients, and preparing meals that are both satisfying to the palate and nourishing. This is a colorful tapestry of flavors meant to improve your wellbeing, not a place for deprivation.

We honor the victories of women over 50 who have adopted intermittent fasting through personal narratives and motivational speeches. They talk about the hardships, successes, and life-changing events that occurred along their own journeys. That proves how strong and resilient you are on the inside.

So, "Intermittent Fasting for Women Over 50" is your reliable guide if you're ready to rethink your relationship with food, accept the wisdom of your body, and set off on a path of self-discovery. Together, let's explore this fascinating territory and realize your potential for a more vibrant, healthy version of yourself. A voyage of nourishing wisdom awaits you!

Chapter 1: Understanding Intermittent Fasting (IF)

What Is Intermittent Fasting?

Intermittent fasting is a lifestyle method that is gaining popularity and recognition; it is a rhythmic dance between periods of eating and fasting that transcends age and helps numerous elements of our well-being. Think of it as a breath of fresh air in the field of nutrition, bringing simplicity to an area that is frequently overrun by intricate diet regimens.

Fundamentally, intermittent fasting has nothing to do with calorie counting or deprivation. It's a flexible approach that encourages people to adopt a more deliberate and mindful eating style. Instead of prescribing particular foods, it emphasizes the timing of meals to align with our bodies' innate cycles.

What precisely is intermittent fasting, then? It is, essentially, the habit of alternately fasting and eating. Intermittent fasting puts more emphasis on when you eat than typical diets, which dictate what you should consume. It's similar to arranging a beautiful symphony in which the intervals between the notes are just as important as the sounds themselves.

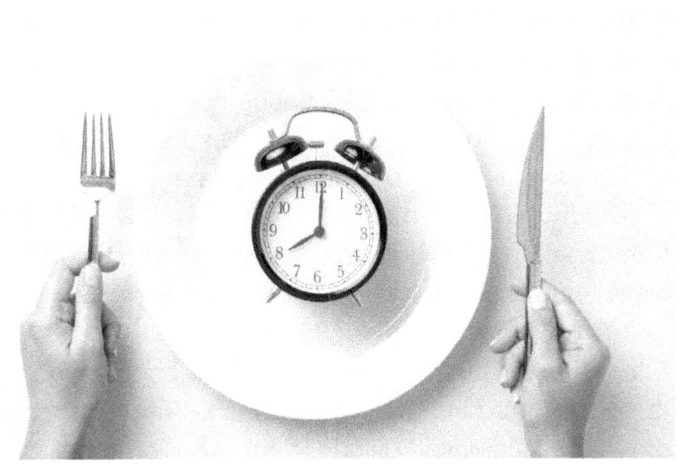

Creating windows of time for eating and then allowing the body to relax from food intake during specified fasting intervals is the main goal of intermittent fasting. It's similar to giving your digestive system a well-earned vacation so it can recharge and work at its best. Its flexibility allows people to select different ways according to their lifestyle, health objectives, and preferences.

The 16/8 strategy is one of the most often used strategies, in which people restrict their daily eating to an 8-hour window and fast for 16 hours. It promotes a natural and intuitive approach of absorbing food within a set timeframe, rather than rigorous meal planning. Imagine it as establishing a regular pattern whereby fasting times are easily incorporated into your schedule without requiring intricate computations.

The 5:2 diet, which calls for eating normally for five days and cutting calories to 25% of the usual amount on two non-consecutive days, is another strategy that is gaining popularity. This method offers a well-balanced framework that fits both excess and moderation within a weekly schedule.

Alternate-day fasting may be ideal for people who want to take a more impromptu approach. With this strategy, days of substantial calorie restriction or total fasting alternate with days of usual eating. This flexible method enables people to align their fasting schedule with their social and leisure obligations.

Another aspect is extended fasting, which involves going longer stretches without eating—often up to a day. Although it may seem overwhelming at first, many people find it surprisingly doable and experience a sense of empowerment as they learn to harness their body's resiliency for adaptation.

Let's now explore the mystery of sporadic fasting. Beyond its apparent simplicity, this exercise has a series of physiological advantages. The body switches from using glucose as its main energy source during fasting periods to using stored fat. This metabolic dance promotes general health by supporting cellular repair mechanisms and helping with weight management.

Furthermore, hormones like growth hormone and insulin are greatly impacted by intermittent fasting, which in turn affects cellular regeneration and repair. It's similar to giving your body a mild tune-up, improving its capacity to flourish and adjust as you go smoothly through various phases of life.

When it comes to aging gracefully, women over 50 can benefit greatly from intermittent fasting. This method responds to the body's changing needs in harmony with hormonal cycles, offering a lasting and natural means of promoting health and vitality.

Essentially, intermittent fasting is a process of self-discovery rather than a strict set of guidelines. It's about creating a healthy relationship with food, letting your body thrive, and accepting a rhythm that suits your own preferences and way of life. Thus, as you set out on this path, think of intermittent fasting as a delightful dance with your body's inherent knowledge rather than as a restricted trip.

Historical Context and Evolution

Finding out about the history and development of intermittent fasting takes us on an interesting trip through time, showing us how this way of eating has become a part of human history. The history of intermittent fasting goes back to many different cultures and societies, each of which adopted the practice for their own unique reasons.

In the past, when our story starts, fasting wasn't just a way to lose weight; it was also often a religious or cultural practice. From the Greeks to the Egyptians, people from many ancient cultures fasted as a way to clean themselves and improve their mental discipline. For instance, in ancient Greece, fasting was considered a way to achieve mental clarity and heightened attention during important philosophical and intellectual pursuits.

Moving forward in our historical exploration, we find intermittent fasting playing a major role in various religious practices. Religions such as Islam, Christianity, and Judaism add fasting into their traditions. During the holy month of Ramadan, Muslims engage in daily fasting from dawn to sunset, a practice that goes back over a millennium. Similarly, Christian fasting traditions during Lent and Jewish fasting on Yom Kippur have deep historical roots.

The Renaissance period saw a shift in the view of fasting, with thinkers like Leonardo da Vinci and Paracelsus contemplating the potential health benefits. Da Vinci, known for his artistic genius, often spoke of the benefits of a moderate and restrained diet, echoing sentiments that align with intermittent fasting principles.

Fast forward to the 20th century, and we meet the groundbreaking work of scientists like Dr. Clive McCay and Dr. Ancel Keys. In the 1930s, Dr. McCay performed landmark research on rats, demonstrating that calorie restriction could extend their lifespan. Dr. Ancel Keys, in the 1940s, performed the Minnesota Starvation Experiment, showing the physiological and psychological effects of severe calorie restriction.

The mid-20th century witnessed the emergence of intermittent fasting as a possible therapeutic tool. Dr. Benjamin Sandler, a prominent physician, advocated for alternate-day fasting as a way to manage certain health conditions. His work laid the foundation for future study into the health benefits of intermittent fasting.

The 21st century marks a resurgence of interest in intermittent fasting, driven not only by scientific research but also by a growing health and wellness movement. With the advent of the internet, knowledge about fasting became more accessible, leading to an increased awareness of its potential benefits. Celebrities, athletes, and health influencers began sharing their positive experiences with intermittent fasting, adding to its popularity.

Scientific study has played a pivotal role in shaping our understanding of intermittent fasting. Studies have proven its effect on insulin sensitivity, metabolic health, and longevity. The discovery of autophagy, the cellular recycling process stimulated during fasting, has further fueled interest in the possible anti-aging effects of intermittent fasting.

As we navigate the historical evolution of intermittent fasting, it's important to recognize the amalgamation of ancient wisdom, religious practices, and scientific advancements that have shaped its trajectory. The story weaves together threads from diverse cultures, historical eras, and scientific breakthroughs, forming a rich tapestry that underscores the enduring relevance and adaptability of intermittent fasting.

In a nutshell the historical journey of intermittent fasting invites us to appreciate its deep roots in human civilization, recognizing it not only as a modern dietary trend but as a practice with a profound and lasting legacy. As we continue to discover its benefits through scientific inquiry, we are reminded that intermittent fasting is not merely a fleeting voyage but a timeless exploration of health and well-being.

Benefits and Risks for Women Over 50

Let's explore the pleasant territory of knowing the benefits as well as any hazards that ladies in this age range might experience

.

Advantages for Women Who Are Over 50

1. Metabolic Magic:

Your metabolism can benefit greatly from adopting an intermittent fasting lifestyle. The slowing of metabolic rates that come with aging frequently results in weight gain. The ability of intermittent fasting to revitalize metabolism can help with weight management and encourage a more favorable body composition.

2. Hormonal Harmony:

Life involves hormonal swings, especially for women over 50. Research has demonstrated the beneficial effects of intermittent fasting on hormones such as insulin and human growth hormone, which in turn leads to an enhanced hormonal equilibrium. Better mood, more energy, and even improved cognitive function can come from this.

3. Brain Boost:

Intermittent fasting has been associated with neuroprotective effects, which is relevant to cognitive performance. Fasting triggers the process of autophagy, which aids in the elimination of damaged cells and promotes the development of new, healthy ones. This may improve general brain health and reduce the risk of neurodegenerative disorders.

4. Inflammation Intervention:

As we become older, chronic inflammation is a prevalent concern and is linked to a number of health problems. The body's natural anti-inflammatory response could be triggered by intermittent fasting, lowering inflammation levels. Thus, there may be a lower chance of developing chronic illnesses and better joint health as a result.

5. Blood Sugar Stabilization:

As we age, maintaining stable blood sugar levels becomes more and more important. By helping to control blood sugar, intermittent fasting may lower the risk of type 2 diabetes. Given the higher risk of insulin resistance in women over 50, this is especially significant at this point in their lives.

6. Heart Health Haven:

Heart health is very important, and your cardiovascular system may benefit from intermittent fasting. Improvements in a number of cardiovascular risk variables, including blood pressure and cholesterol, have been linked to it. This may help maintain a healthier heart, in addition to other benefits related to weight management.

Risks

1. Nutritional Requirements:

Even though there are several advantages to intermittent fasting, it's important to make sure you're still getting enough nutrients. For healthy bones, women over 50 require certain minerals, like calcium and vitamin D. It is crucial to monitor nutrient intake during meal periods in order to promote general health.

2. Hormonal Factors to Consider:

The menopausal hormone shifts can affect the body's reaction to fasting. It's critical to pay attention to your body and modify your fasting schedule as necessary. Speaking with a medical expert can offer tailored advice and make sure that intermittent fasting is compatible with your hormone profile.

3. Levels of Energy

While many people find that intermittent fasting increases their energy levels, some women may find it difficult at first to adjust to this eating schedule. It's critical to listen to your body's cues and modify as necessary. Try a variety of fasting techniques and meal times to see what suits you the best.

4. Possible Stress:

The body may experience some stress from intermittent fasting, particularly if it is not done carefully. It is critical for women over 50 to manage their stress. Incorporating stress-relieving techniques like meditation or mild exercise can enhance intermittent fasting and advance general health.

In conclusion, women over 50 who want to practice intermittent fasting are embarking on a complex journey that is full of possible benefits and considerations. By adopting a conscious strategy, being acutely aware of your body's cues, and maybe having a cordial discussion with your doctor, you may confidently navigate these waters and maximize the advantages of your lifestyle decision while lowering the risks. To a bright and well-traveling journey!

How It Differs from Traditional Diets

Traditional diets often recommend three meals a day, along with snacks, creating a recognizable pattern that is passed down through the generations. These diets' basic tenet is a steady intake of calories distributed equally throughout the awake hours. Breakfast, lunch, and dinner follow a set pattern, never straying from the predetermined plot. It's a planned narrative.

By changing the timing of meals, intermittent fasting, on the other hand, offers a dynamic plot and subverts the traditional narrative. Intermittent fasting encourages a period of deliberate abstinence as opposed to a continuous intake of calories throughout the day, resulting in an enticing cycle of eating and fasting. Similar to a thrilling plot twist, this narrative shift carefully introduces and withholds characters (nutrients) for maximum effect.

The idea of timing is one of the most important differences. Traditional diets place a strong emphasis on eating regular meals at set times, with breakfast being seen as the most important meal of the day. On the other hand, intermittent fasting alters the temporal terrain and promotes a more adaptable schedule for meals. During times of fasting, the food becomes purposefully interrupted, enabling the body to use stored energy and start cellular cleaning processes like autophagy.

The ways in which these two dietary approaches tackle metabolism also diverge in their storytelling techniques. Traditional diets keep the metabolic engine operating at a constant speed by supplying an even amount of calories. But because intermittent fasting alternates between feeding and fasting states, it adds a degree of unpredictableness. This change may cause a mental shock to the metabolism, causing it to adjust and optimize energy use in response to sporadic fuel supply.

The story of intermittent fasting's effects on hormone regulation may be the most convincing one. Traditional diets hardly address the complex hormonal orchestra that governs our health. But in this context, intermittent fasting really shines, causing a symphony of hormonal shifts. During fasting times, there is an improvement in insulin sensitivity that helps with blood sugar regulation. There is also an increase in growth hormone production that helps with fat utilization and muscle maintenance.

Moreover, the storyline of intermittent fasting goes beyond the material world and explores people's psychological connections to food. It's possible that traditional diets unintentionally promote limitation by dividing items into "allowed" and "forbidden" categories. Because of its rhythmic approach, intermittent fasting encourages a more intuitive and free mindset when it comes to eating. It's a narrative that allows people to enjoy their food without having to worry about continual dietary monitoring.

Essentially, the story of how intermittent fasting varies from traditional diets is one of flexibility, unexpected discoveries, and a sophisticated comprehension of the body's requirements. It's a story that questions the status quo, encouraging readers to reconsider how they relate to food and to embrace a worldview in which purposeful fasting leads to a more lively and healthy existence. Thus, keep in mind that the beauty of these nutritional pages is not only in their distinctions but also in the capacity for personal growth that each strategy offers.

CHAPTER 2: Physiology of Intermittent Fasting

Impact on Metabolism

A world of opportunities arises from intermittent fasting, particularly with its tremendous effect on metabolism. Now let's explore the details of how this strategy affects the body's complex metabolic dance and learn the science underlying the alterations that occur.

Fundamentally, metabolism is the complex network of metabolic reactions that powers our bodies. See it as a vibrant symphony in which every instrument is vital to the overall harmony. Rather than upsetting this harmony, intermittent fasting adds a new beat that produces a song of health advantages.

Insulin is a major instrument in this metabolic orchestra. Our bodies release insulin when we eat, particularly when it comes to carbs, which aids cells in absorbing glucose for energy. By setting aside specific times for eating and fasting, intermittent fasting helps to regulate the synthesis of insulin more evenly. This may improve insulin sensitivity, which is important for controlling weight and preventing type 2 diabetes.

Furthermore, intermittent fasting is a metabolic dance that goes beyond insulin regulation. The body uses alternative energy sources—most notably, stored fat—during the fasting window. This process, called ketosis, promotes the body's and brain's conversion of fat into ketones, an additional energy source. Because of this, those who practice intermittent fasting might be able to burn fat more efficiently, which would help them lose weight and have a better body composition.

In addition to its physiological effects, intermittent fasting affects the metabolic rate via encouraging autophagy. Think of it as a cleanup staff for cells. Cells undergo a process called autophagy, which helps them recycle and eliminate damaged components to encourage cellular renewal. Intermittent fasting may increase cellular resilience and longevity by promoting this self-healing process.

The complex relationships between metabolic health and circadian rhythms—internal body clocks that govern a range of physiological functions—are profound. By better synchronizing meal timing with the body's internal clock, intermittent fasting optimizes the metabolic dance in accordance with these inherent cycles. Overall health and metabolic efficiency may be improved by this alignment.

Furthermore, the body experiences a minor degree of stress during intermittent fasting. Despite its negative connotations, stress can be advantageous when used moderately and occasionally. Hormesis is the idea that stress causes the body to adapt and become stronger.

Intermittent fasting has the potential to protect against a range of age-related disorders by inducing the creation of heat shock proteins and antioxidant defenses through hormesis.

Think about fasting intermittently as a metabolic workout. Intermittent fasting fortifies and challenges your metabolic systems, much like physical exercise challenges and strengthens your muscles. It's a metabolic symphony training program that enhances resilience, adaptability, and peak performance in your body.

It is noteworthy that intermittent fasting is not a universally applicable treatment, even though it can serve as a transforming conductor in the metabolic orchestra. When starting this trip, things like age, personal health issues, and lifestyle should be taken into account. Getting advice from nutritionists or medical specialists can assist customize an intermittent fasting plan that fits well with each person's needs and objectives.

The effects of intermittent fasting on metabolism provide an enthralling window into the complex musical composition that is the human body. Through comprehension of the subtleties involved in this metabolic dance, people can use its potential advantages, cultivating a more robust and healthy ensemble that contributes to overall well-being. Let the metabolic song begin as you enter the realm of intermittent fasting, and may your health enjoy the harmonizing benefits.

Hormonal Changes

The significant influence of this lifestyle shift on hormonal shifts, which leads to a comprehensive alteration in our bodies' functioning, is one of its intriguing features.

Hormonal changes become a defining feature of aging in women. But intermittent fasting has a special effect on these hormonal shifts and provides a novel way to welcome the golden years full of vitality.

Insulin is one of the main hormones impacted by periodic fasting. This hormone, which controls blood sugar levels, changes in a good way when fasting occurs. Insulin sensitivity increases in women over 50 who intermittently fast, which helps them better control their blood sugar levels. By doing this, you lower your chance of getting type 2 diabetes while also improving your metabolic health in general.

Growth hormone is another important instrument in the hormonal symphony. Growth hormone levels usually decrease with age and are often linked to youth and energy. On the other hand, intermittent fasting orchestrates an increase in growth hormone production like a conductor. This hormone surge helps women deal with the complexities of aging by promoting fat metabolism, maintaining muscular mass, and even helping to maintain bone density.

Intermittent fasting also modifies the thyroid, an important organ that controls metabolism. Fasting may initially lower thyroid hormone levels, according to certain research, but over time, the body adjusts and thyroid function returns to normal. In order to fully benefit from intermittent fasting, consistency and patience are essential, as demonstrated by the delicate tango between thyroid health and fasting.

During menopause, estrogen—a hormone essential to women's health—changes. Surprisingly, intermittent fasting may provide some comfort through altering estrogen levels. According to some research, women who practice intermittent fasting may experience a reduction in estrogen levels, which could help to regulate hormones and potentially lessen the symptoms of hormonal imbalances.

The stress hormone cortisol also comes into focus while discussing intermittent fasting. Although there are concerns that fasting could increase cortisol levels, research shows that intermittent fasting does not always result in chronic stress under controlled conditions. Rather, over time, the body adjusts and becomes more stress-resistant.

Known as the hunger hormones, leptin and ghrelin perform a unique dance when a person fasts intermittently. These hormones achieve a harmonic balance when the body adapts to new eating habits, which aids women in better understanding and controlling their hunger signals.

The hormonal stage is dynamic and complex in the vast spectacle of intermittent fasting. The total synergy that improves the health and well-being of women over 50 is just as beautiful as the changes themselves. It's like having a cordial discussion with your body, a little prod in the direction of a more vibrant, healthy self. Therefore, keep in mind that intermittent fasting is a celebration of wellbeing at any age rather than merely a fad while you navigate the ups and downs of these hormonal shifts.

Cellular Repair and Autophagy

Within the intriguing realm of intermittent fasting, the processes of autophagy and cellular repair emerge as key players in enhancing general health. Don't be intimidated by the technical terminology; instead, consider it as your body's internal repair team, working nonstop to keep everything in perfect condition.

Consider your cells as minuscule, industrious machines that generate energy, mend damage, and keep your body in balance. These factories can begin to show symptoms of wear and tear as we become older. This is where the amazing process of autophagy is triggered by intermittent fasting, acting like a superhero.

Your body uses autophagy, which is derived from the Greek words "auto" (self) and "phagy" (to eat), as a sort of internal house cleaning. Your body goes into a state during intermittent fasting, particularly during the fasting periods, where it is more intent on eliminating the cellular components that are aging, damaged, or not performing well. It's similar to dispatching a group of specialists to find and recycle anything that isn't operating at its best.

Imagine that your cells are going through a thorough cleansing procedure while you enjoy your green tea during a period of fasting. Defunct proteins, worn-out organelles, and other cellular detritus are the targets of autophagy. Your body breaks these components down into new, healthier cell structures rather than allowing them to build up and perhaps cause issues.

The benefits of cellular regeneration for your health are real and not simply theoretical. According to research, autophagy may be essential in preventing a number of age-related illnesses, such as cancer and neurological diseases. Intermittent fasting ultimately aids in the maintenance of a cleaner, more efficient system within your body by encouraging the clearance of damaged cells.

Furthermore, there is a close connection between autophagy and longevity. You're essentially allowing your body to age more gracefully by improving the quality of your cells and lessening the load of damaged components.

Let's now discuss cellular repair. Your body devotes resources to repair processes during fasting times, when it's not occupied with breaking down food. This repair process involves strengthening cellular integrity and repairing damage to DNA. It's as if your body is saying, "Leave everything in perfect working order, we've got a moment of downtime."

Your body's repair mechanisms are triggered by intermittent fasting, which results in a harmonious symphony of renewal. Better cellular repair can strengthen your immune system and make you more capable of warding off infections in addition to making your body more resilient.

Essentially, intermittent fasting becomes a comprehensive approach to health, with an emphasis on how your body renews itself rather than just what you consume. Thus, the next time you choose to observe a fasting window, remember that you are actively engaging in a cellular rejuvenation process that improves your general health and wellbeing in addition to simply refraining from eating.

Adapting to Aging

The years pile up nicely, and our bodies alter in a hundred different ways. Accepting the idea of intermittent fasting requires a special adjustment to the unavoidable aging process, especially for women over 50. Imagine it not as a huge obstacle but rather as a dance with time, a rhythmic dance that enables you to appreciate the beauty of every instant that passes.

Understanding the physiological changes associated with aging is crucial throughout this stage of life. Sometimes referred to as the body's engine, metabolism might slow down. Although it's a normal part of the process, intermittent fasting turns into a helpful ally. It stimulates a healthy metabolism and helps your body use energy more effectively.

Another complex thread in the aging puzzle is hormonal changes. The subtle guidance provided by intermittent fasting aids in the preservation of hormonal homeostasis. This can be especially important for women over 50 because this is a time when progesterone and estrogen swings are typical. By helping to stabilize these hormones, fasting promotes general health and vigor.

Customization is key in the process of adjusting to age via intermittent fasting. It's about adjusting your strategy to your particular requirements and tastes. It becomes crucial to take into account your unique lifestyle, eating preferences, and state of health. There isn't one approach that works for everyone; instead, you should create a strategy that matches your unique needs and makes the process fun.

While aging may be difficult to navigate, intermittent fasting offers a useful compass. It becomes an art to take care of your nutritional needs, balancing your intake of vital nutrients to meet your body's evolving needs. It's about enjoying meals rich in nutrients that feed your body and spirit and provide a symphony of flavors that your tongue will love.

Controlling urges and hunger turns into a mental dance. You can learn to accept hunger as a normal part of the process by engaging in intermittent fasting. It's about approaching food mindfully, not about deprivation. We recognize and accommodate cravings, those irrational impulses for particular meals. By putting more emphasis on contentment than mere consumption, fasting becomes a strategy for creating a healthier relationship with food.

Exercise is a key element in aging well and is frequently regarded as essential to a healthy lifestyle. It's about a mild, customized routine that fits your age and physical level rather than intense workouts. When coordinated well, intermittent fasting and exercise can complement one another and promote general health.

As on any journey through life, health issues could surface. Because intermittent fasting is flexible, it promotes speaking with medical professionals. It's important to be aware of any pre-existing illnesses and to collaborate in order to make sure that your fasting strategy supports your overall health objectives.

Adjusting to aging through intermittent fasting is a dynamic process that involves a cordial dialogue with your body as it ages gracefully. It's about accepting life's ups and downs, recognizing the shifts, and discovering a beat that suits your own melody. With time, intermittent fasting in this amiable dance with age transforms from a tactic into a wonderful traveling partner.

CHAPTER 3: Tailoring Intermittent Fasting for Women Over 50

Addressing Nutritional Needs

Our bodies experience little changes as the years pass, and our nutritional needs also do. Adopting intermittent fasting entails thinking about what your body actually requires in addition to changing when you eat. Now, let's explore the topic of dietary advice for the amazing person over 50!

Let's start by talking about protein, which is your diet's unsung hero. It's for everyone who wants to sustain overall health and muscular mass, not only bodybuilders. Since our bodies become less adept at utilizing protein as we age, it is imperative that you include a sufficient amount of foods high in protein throughout your meals. Lean meats, dairy products, legumes, and nuts are your friends when it comes to protein.

Let's now highlight the importance of healthy fats. You read correctly—fats may be both delicious and healthful! Choose heart-healthy foods like fatty salmon, avocados, and olive oil to give your body the critical fatty acids it needs to promote heart and brain function. Invite these fats to your plate; they're like the members of your nutritious entourage.

Remember the unsung heroes of nutrition: minerals and vitamins. The secret to opening up different body functions is found in these tiny powerhouses. For example, as bone health becomes more important as we age, calcium becomes increasingly more important. Include dairy, leafy greens, and fortified foods in your diet to make sure your bones are receiving the care they require.

Let's dispel a common misconception regarding carbohydrates: they are not harmful. Choose complex carbs to keep you full during your fasting window, such as whole grains, fruits, and vegetables. These nutrient-dense carbohydrates are your go-to friends since they keep you full and prepared for anything life throws at you.

Another essential component of this nutritional symphony is hydration. Not only does water help you stay hydrated, but it is also necessary for proper digestion, nutritional absorption, and general body functions. Throughout the day, make a conscious effort to consume water to keep your body hydrated and aid in the fasting process.

When you go out on your adventure of intermittent fasting, visualize your nutritional palette as the vibrant variety of fruits and vegetables. Because of their abundance in fiber, vitamins, and antioxidants, they promote general health and make fasting easier.

Your guide to this dietary journey is balance. A well-rounded diet should consist of a range of foods to ensure that you are meeting the specific needs of your body. Pay attention to your body's cues, try out a variety of meals, and identify the combo that leaves you feeling full and alive.

As you customize your intermittent fasting regimen, keep in mind that proper nutrition for your body involves consuming the right foods at the right times rather than merely eating when you feel like it. Think of your dietary requirements as a daily letter of love and care to yourself, one that will help you stay youthful and radiant.

Adapting to Individual Lifestyles

One size does not fit all when it comes to intermittent fasting; it's more like choosing a fitted suit that exactly matches your own style. Choosing to adopt intermittent fasting for women over 50 is about creating a plan that works with your unique lifestyle, not about following strict guidelines.

Let's explore how incorporating intermittent fasting into your daily routine might be harmonious. Think of it as a helpful buddy that adjusts to your tastes so that the road to greater health flows naturally into your daily schedule.

Prioritize your daily schedule above all else. If you're the type of person who prefers to eat breakfast first thing in the morning, the 16/8 technique may be right for you. This method makes it simple to adapt into your natural rhythm by limiting your eating window to 8 hours and fasting for 16 hours. But worry not, night owls: you can modify your eating window to better accommodate your nocturnal tendencies because there is flexibility in the fasting cosmos.

Let's now discuss those among us who are social butterflies. Fasting intermittently doesn't have to be done alone; it may be easily incorporated into get-togethers and family meals. Select a fasting technique that fits in with your social schedule. With its two non-consecutive days of intermittent calorie restriction, the 5:2 diet gives you the flexibility to indulge on special occasions while adhering to a set fasting schedule.

Those with erratic schedules or unforeseen obligations may find the alternate-day fasting method to be a lifesaver. You can freely modify your calorie intake on fasting days according to your energy requirements. As promised, it's a dance-free method for keeping consistency while adjusting to the ups and downs of life's responsibilities.

Take into account your own dietary choices as well. Breaking your fast with a hearty morning meal is totally appropriate if you're a breakfast aficionado. Similarly, if you are excited about enjoying a substantial supper, merely modify your eating window. The flexibility of intermittent fasting to suit your food preferences is its greatest asset.

Let's now talk about the fitness enthusiasts that love being active. Exercise and fasting can complement one another and improve general well being. Make sure you adjust your fasting schedule to fit your exercise regimen so that you can fuel your physical activities.

Recall that intermittent fasting is a framework that is flexible enough to fit your lifestyle rather than a strict one. Instead of seeing it as a hardship, see it as a chance to establish a fun and long-lasting practice that improves your health and energy. The secret is to seize the opportunities it presents and customize it to suit your needs, developing a customized strategy that becomes second nature and blends in perfectly with your everyday routine.

Potential Challenges and Solutions

It might be difficult to navigate the route of intermittent fasting, particularly for women over 50. Accepting this shift in lifestyle calls for a combination of perseverance, patience, and adaptability. Let's discuss several possible roadblocks and their potential fixes to help your intermittent fasting experience go more smoothly.

The Timing Dilemma

Finding the ideal fasting window that fits with one's lifestyle can be a struggle for many people. It might be challenging to develop a regular fasting schedule when juggling obligations to your family, job, and social life. Here, adaptability is the answer. Try a variety of fasting hours to see what works best for you. Finding a sustainable routine that fits your daily life is more important than following strict guidelines.

Handling the Pangs of Hunger

An inevitable side effect of fasting is hunger, which can be intimidating at first. See hunger as a comrade on your path to wellbeing rather than as an enemy. Consider progressively extending your fasting window, drinking plenty of water, and include foods high in fiber in your meals to help reduce hunger pangs. Over time, these techniques can assist you in developing resistance to cravings.

Social Coercion and Get-togethers

It can be difficult to attend family get-togethers or social activities when everyone else is eating. Don't worry; this is your chance to demonstrate how flexible your intermittent fasting lifestyle is. Tell your loved ones about your objectives, and they might surprise you by making encouraging changes to your meal plans. To ensure you don't feel left out and can stay on track, bring your own wholesome food to share.

Levels of Energy and Fatigue

Energy swings are possible for certain people, particularly in the early stages of intermittent fasting. During your eating window, concentrate on consuming foods high in nutrients to offset this. Including lean proteins, healthy fats, and complex carbohydrates will help you feel energized all day. Additionally, pay attention to your body. If you have weariness, think about modifying your fasting hours or consulting a medical practitioner.

Emotional Cues for Overeating

We often find that our connection with food is heavily influenced by our emotions. It's critical to identify emotional triggers and develop other coping strategies. For emotional support, take part in things you enjoy, practice mindfulness, or get in touch with friends. You may empower yourself to make better decisions and have a positive relationship with food by addressing emotional eating.

Peaking Development

Sometimes people hit a wall when trying to lose weight or achieve other health-related objectives. This stage is typical of a lot of wellness journeys. Celebrate non-scale wins like increased energy, better sleep, or increased mental clarity rather than giving up. If losing weight is your main objective, review your eating patterns and think about getting advice from a nutritionist for individualized advice.

Changes in Hormone Levels

Hormonal changes can affect women's experiences with intermittent fasting, particularly those over 50. Pay attention to the cues your body gives you and modify your fasting schedule as necessary. If you discover that some days of the month are harder for you than others, think about taking a more accommodating stance on those days. Make self-care a priority and pay attention to your body's demands in order to stay in balance.Overcoming the difficulties of intermittent fasting is essentially a path of self-awareness and adaptability. Treat yourself with care as you accept the process. There's no one-size-fits-all answer; instead, you need to figure out what works best for you. You learn important lessons from every obstacle that enhance your general wellbeing.

CHAPTER 4: Popular Intermittent Fasting Methods

16/8 Method

The 16/8 method becomes well-known and approachable, creating waves in the movement towards a healthy way of living. This approach, which is based on adaptability and simplicity, has a lot of potential, particularly for people who want balance and wellbeing in their daily lives.

	Day 1	Day 2	Day 3	Day 4	Day 5	Day 6	Day 7
Midnight	FAST	FAST	FAST	FAST	FAST	FAST	FAST
4am	FAST	FAST	FAST	FAST	FAST	FAST	FAST
8am	FAST	FAST	FAST	FAST	FAST	FAST	FAST
12pm	First Meal	First Meal	First Meal	First Meal	First Meal	First Meal	First Meal
4pm	Last Meal by 8pm	Last Meal by 8pm	Last Meal by 8pm	Last Meal by 8pm	Last Meal by 8pm	Last Meal by 8pm	Last Meal by 8pm
8pm	FAST	FAST	FAST	FAST	FAST	FAST	FAST
Midnight	FAST	FAST	FAST	FAST	FAST	FAST	FAST

Imagine living in a world where you are not restricted by a rigid diet and can still enjoy your favorite foods. That is precisely what the 16/8 approach permits, giving you an 8-hour window during which to eat and 16 hours during which to fast. Instead of focusing on deprivation, redefine when you take in your nourishment.

Adopting the 16/8 approach offers a novel viewpoint on mealtimes. Say good-bye to the traditional three-meal-a-day schedule and embrace the concept of narrowing your eating window to a shorter time frame. Imagine enjoying your breakfast, lunch, and dinner all in the allotted eight hours, and letting your body recover and replenish itself during the fasting period.

The flexibility of the 16/8 technique to suit different lifestyles is one of its most notable qualities. This technique can be adjusted to fit your daily schedule, regardless of whether you're a night owl or an early riser. It fits into a variety of schedules with ease, giving you the flexibility to select the hours that work best for your eating window.

Furthermore, the 16/8 method's simplicity doesn't require you to change your eating habits. You can enjoy your meals and still profit from intermittent fasting, as there is opportunity for flexibility and enjoyment. Optimizing when you eat is more important than limiting what you eat.

Looking more closely at the physiological side of things, the 16/8 technique uses the body's circadian rhythm. This is consistent with our circadian rhythm, which may accelerate metabolism during the window of opportunity for feeding. Your body may use nutrients more effectively as it adjusts to this pattern, resulting in increased energy and general wellbeing.

The advantages of the 16/8 technique go beyond managing weight. Studies indicate that it may facilitate improved regulation of blood sugar and enhance cardiovascular well-being. Letting the body fast for longer periods of time may help improve cellular repair mechanisms and lower inflammation, both of which are beneficial to long-term health.

You don't have to go through this journey alone if you choose to use the 16/8 technique. To help with the adjustment, there are many online communities and forums filled with advice, recipe ideas, and experiences from others. Speaking with people who are following a similar route might inspire you and give you a sense of support as you investigate the many facets of this intermittent fasting technique.

It's critical to approach the 16/8 method with the knowledge that each person is different. Pay attention to your body's signals, listen to it, and modify as necessary. Part of the procedure is experimenting to determine the rhythm that best fits your lifestyle and health objectives.

To sum up, the 16/8 technique encourages a comprehensive approach to wellbeing rather than merely providing an eating schedule. Accept the flexibility, eat with awareness, and allow this technique to become a natural part of your daily routine. The 16/8 technique invites you to take a journey toward a more balanced and healthy version of yourself because of its welcoming and adjustable nature.

5:2 Diet

Adopting a new lifestyle can be exhilarating as well as intimidating, particularly when it involves changing how we think about eating. The 5:2 diet, often known as the "Fast Diet," is a well-liked intermittent fasting technique that draws attention while offering a flexible and well-balanced approach to weight control for individuals of all ages.

DAY 1	DAY 2	DAY 3	DAY 4	DAY 5	DAY 6	DAY 7
Eat Normally	Women: 500 Calories	Eat normally	Eat normally	Women: 500 Calories	Eat normally	Eat normally

Unveiling the 5:2 Diet

Imagine following a diet that promotes a distinctive eating pattern rather than limiting your access to your daily favorite meals. That's the basic idea behind the 5:2 diet, which is eating in a typical manner for five days a week and then cutting calories on the other two non-consecutive days. Its versatility makes it doable for a broad spectrum of people, including those who are over 50.

How It Works

There's no need to track every calorie or stay away from certain food groups on the five usual eating days. Rather, it pertains to upholding a nutritious, well-balanced diet. The two days of fasting are the most interesting aspects. Calorie consumption is limited on these days; for women, this usually translates to 500–600 calories. It is thought that this sporadic calorie restriction will lead to a number of health advantages, such as enhanced metabolic health and weight loss.

Tailored for Women Over 50

The 5:2 diet's adaptability to various age groups is one of its notable features, which makes it especially tempting for women over 50. It becomes increasingly important to discover a sustainable strategy for keeping a healthy weight as we age since our bodies change. This is addressed by the 5:2 diet, which provides a flexible framework that can be modified to suit different dietary requirements and lifestyles.

Health Benefits Beyond Weight Loss

Although losing weight is a major benefit, the 5:2 diet aims to achieve more than just weight loss. According to research, there are a number of health advantages to intermittent fasting, including decreased inflammation, increased brain function, and improved insulin sensitivity. These potential benefits go beyond the physical for women over 50, providing a comprehensive approach to wellbeing.

Navigating the Fasting Days

Although many people find that the fasting days are difficult at first, they may be easily managed with enough preparation. Minimizing hunger pangs can be achieved by eating a diet high in nutrients and distributing a few calories throughout the day. It's also critical to drink enough water and pay attention to your body, making any necessary adjustments. It's not about deprivation but about mindfully consuming less on certain days.

Realistic and Sustainable

The 5:2 diet is unique since it is realistic and long-term. It promotes a long-term, balanced approach as opposed to quick fixes or the total removal of certain food groups. This makes it a good choice for women over 50 who want to make a long-term lifestyle adjustment that works.

Conclusion

Women over 50 are invited to adopt a flexible and pleasurable approach to health management by embracing the 5:2 diet. Eating is important more than simply what you eat; it's also about timing your meals to fit into your lifestyle. Thus, if you're seeking for a flexible and amiable approach to health, the 5:2 diet may be the encouraging friend you've been waiting for.

Alternate-Day Fasting

DAY1	DAY 2	DAY 3	DAY 4	DAY 5	DAY 6	DAY 7
Eat Normally	24- hour fast Or Eats only a few hundred calories	Eat normally	24- hour fast Or Eats only a few hundred calories	Eat normally	24- hour fast Or Eats only a few hundred calories	Eat normally

In the world of intermittent fasting, one approach that has gained significant attention is Alternate-Day Fasting (ADF). It's not just a diet; it's a lifestyle that offers a refreshing twist to conventional eating patterns. Let's delve into the essence of Alternate-Day Fasting and explore how it could be your ticket to a healthier and more balanced life.

Imagine a routine where you savor your favorite meals without feeling confined by strict dietary rules every day. Alternate-Day Fasting allows you to do just that. On fasting days, you consume a significantly reduced number of calories or even abstain from food altogether, while on non-fasting days, you indulge in a more typical eating pattern. It's a rhythm that aligns with your body's natural ebb and flow, offering a sustainable way to manage weight and improve overall well-being.

One of the key advantages of Alternate-Day Fasting is its adaptability. Whether you're a newcomer to intermittent fasting or a seasoned practitioner, this method can be tailored to suit your preferences and lifestyle. It provides the flexibility to choose fasting days based on your schedule, making it a feasible option for women over 50 who are navigating the demands of daily life.

Scientifically, Alternate-Day Fasting triggers various metabolic changes in the body. On fasting days, the body shifts into a state of ketosis, where it relies on stored fat for energy. This not only supports weight loss but also enhances metabolic efficiency. Additionally, research suggests that ADF may have positive effects on cardiovascular health, insulin sensitivity, and inflammation levels.

Beyond the physiological benefits, Alternate-Day Fasting has a remarkable impact on our relationship with food. By embracing a cyclical approach to eating, individuals often find themselves savoring and appreciating their meals more. It fosters a mindful connection with food, steering away from the often stressful and restrictive mindset associated with traditional diets.

Navigating the fasting and non-fasting days may initially present a challenge, but many find that the routine becomes more intuitive over time. It encourages a deeper understanding of hunger cues and allows for a more attuned response to the body's needs. This aspect makes Alternate-Day Fasting not just a dietary strategy but a holistic approach to well-being.

For women over 50, the adaptability of Alternate-Day Fasting can be particularly appealing. It accommodates the diverse nutritional requirements that may come with age, providing a framework that supports health without sacrificing the joy of eating. Moreover, the intermittent nature of ADF can be gentler on the body, offering a sustainable path to maintaining a healthy weight and promoting longevity.

As with any lifestyle change, it's crucial to approach Alternate-Day Fasting with mindfulness and balance. Listening to your body, staying hydrated, and ensuring nutrient-dense meals on non-fasting days are key elements of a successful ADF journey. Consulting with healthcare professionals before embarking on this adventure is always recommended, especially for those with pre-existing health conditions.

In conclusion, Alternate-Day Fasting is not just a trend but a versatile and engaging approach to wellness. It's an invitation to rediscover the joy of eating while promoting health and longevity.

Extended Fasting

Starting a long-term fast can have a profoundly transforming effect on your body and psyche. It's a path toward improved health and wellbeing, not just about going without meals for a long time.

Within the context of fasting, the notion of extended fasting refers to a prolonged period of not eating—usually longer than twenty-four hours. Even while it could seem difficult at first, many people have discovered that implementing prolonged fasting into their lives has tremendous advantages.

The ability of prolonged fasting to stimulate autophagy—the body's natural process of cellular repair—is one of its main benefits. Your body turns its attention from digestion to repair while you fast, dissolving damaged cells and removing waste products from the cell. This revitalizing procedure encourages longevity and general well-being and is similar to pressing the reset button for your body.

Another area where prolonged fasting might have a big influence is weight management. After the first few phases of fasting, your body uses its fat reserves as a source of energy, which promotes fat loss. This metabolic shift may help support a healthier and more long-term strategy for managing weight.

Furthermore, prolonged fasting has demonstrated potential in enhancing insulin sensitivity. Improved insulin use by the body can help control blood sugar levels and lower the risk of type 2 diabetes. As insulin sensitivity tends to decrease with age, this is especially important for people over 50.

Long-term fasting's benefits for the brain are now drawing interest. According to certain research, fasting intervals may improve brain health and guard against age-related neurodegenerative illnesses. Fasting is associated with enhanced mental clarity and attention in many people, demonstrating the complex relationship between gut and brain health.

It is imperative to approach prolonged fasting mindfully and gradually. Start with shorter periods for fasting, like 24 hours, so that your body can adjust and you can better understand how comfortable you are. You can experiment with longer periods of fasting as you grow more accustomed to it, always listening to your body's cues and seeking medical advice as necessary.

In order to maintain your body throughout an extended fast, you must stay hydrated. Black coffee, herbal teas, and water can all help keep electrolyte balance and reduce appetite. But, especially if you're new to fasting, it's crucial to pay attention to your body and avoid pushing yourself too far.

A joyful and sustainable extended fasting journey can be achieved through social support and shared experiences. Making a connection with a group of people who have similar objectives and life experiences can offer support, advice, and a feeling of oneness. Support organizations, internet forums, or simply people who share a similar interest in fasting can provide insightful information and inspiration.

In summary, prolonged fasting is a holistic approach to health that goes beyond a simple physical cleanse. Numerous advantages for your body and mind can be unlocked by embracing this exercise with an open and welcoming mindset. Recall that making the intentional decision to feed your body differently and start down the path to better health and vitality is what matters, not deprivation.

CHAPTER 5: Designing a Personalized Fasting Plan

Assessing Health and Fitness Levels

Starting an intermittent fasting (IF) journey is an exciting step toward improved fitness and health. In order to customize IF to your specific requirements and goals, it's imperative to evaluate your present state of health and fitness before committing to this lifestyle.

First, think about making an appointment for a check-up with your doctor. In addition to ensuring that you're physically ready for intermittent fasting, a thorough health evaluation helps uncover any underlying medical issues. Your physician can offer you advice on cardiovascular fitness, metabolic health, and any specific medical concerns that might affect how you approach intermittent fasting.

Just as crucial is knowing where your fitness level is in the beginning. Choosing the best IF technique and adding the right workouts will be guided by your evaluation of your physical capabilities. Pay attention to your strength, flexibility, and endurance because these attributes affect your total fitness.

Next, assess your nutritional level and eating habits at the moment. Do you currently eat a balanced diet, or could you do better? To learn more about your eating habits, try maintaining a food journal for a few days. This can assist you in determining areas that could require modification so that you can make sure your body is receiving enough nutrition during fasting periods.

Make a note of any current medical issues or drugs you're taking while you evaluate your fitness and health. Your IF schedule may need to be adjusted for certain health conditions, and the timing of your fasting periods may be affected by certain drugs. Talk about these factors with your physician to develop a fasting plan that enhances your general health.

Knowing how stressed you are is another important factor. Persistent stress may affect how your body reacts to fasting, which could impede your progress. Including stress-relieving activities in your intermittent fasting regimen, such meditation or long walks, can improve your general health and effectiveness.

Think about how you sleep as well. Good sleep is essential for general health and can affect your ability to follow an IF regimen. Evaluate the length and quality of your sleep at the moment, and if needed, look into ways to enhance your sleep hygiene. Resting enough aids in your body's ability to heal and adjust to the modifications that intermittent fasting brings about.

Think about how you feel about yourself emotionally and how you view fitness and health. Throughout your journey of intermittent fasting, you will gain power by cultivating a good mindset and a realistic approach. Recognize your objectives and driving forces, and acknowledge minor accomplishments along the route.

Setting reasonable objectives is the next step after evaluating your current state of health and fitness. Setting specific, attainable goals will help you make the most of your intermittent fasting experience, whether your goal is to lose weight, increase energy, or improve your general wellbeing. Recall that development happens gradually, and maintaining a patient and optimistic outlook is essential.

To sum up, the first step to a successful and customized approach to intermittent fasting is to evaluate your current state of health and fitness before beginning. Knowing your body, eliminating any obstacles, and establishing reasonable objectives can help you be ready to start this life-changing path to improved health and vitality.

Setting Realistic Goals

Above all, it's critical to understand that there isn't one intermittent fasting strategy that works for everyone. Consider your particular situation, state of health, and personal preferences as you start. Understanding your own body and matching your goals with attainable milestones are the first steps towards setting realistic goals.

Set a reasonable window for fasting to start. A progressive approach is frequently the most effective for novices. Begin with a short fast, say 12 hours, and then as your body gets used to it, progressively increase it. Your metabolism and digestive system can adjust using this strategy, which lessens the chance of feeling overwhelmed or demoralized.

When creating goals for fasting, take your lifestyle and daily routine into account. It can be more sensible to pick a fasting window that works well with your everyday routine if you have a hectic schedule. In this manner, fasting ceases to be an extra source of stress and instead becomes a normal part of your schedule.

Concentrating on the caliber of your meals throughout eating windows is an additional essential component of goal-setting for intermittent fasting. Make an emphasis on nutrient-dense foods that fuel your body instead of obsessing over calorie counting. Try to maintain a good balance of carbohydrates, healthy fats, and proteins to support your energy and general well-being.

Staying hydrated is essential for IF success. Make it your mission to drink enough water during the fasting period. Drinks like water, herbal teas, and black coffee are great ways to stay hydrated and prevent hunger.

Pay attention to your body. Realistic goal-setting entails recognizing your own signals and making necessary adjustments. Be willing to make adjustments to your strategy if you discover that a specific fasting window is too uncomfortable or interfering with your regular routine. The secret to long-term success with intermittent fasting is flexibility.

Rejoice in non-scale accomplishments. Even though many people may have weight loss as a goal, it's important to recognize other positive changes. Notable successes that support a generally healthy lifestyle include more energy, more mental clarity, and better sleep. Acknowledging these successes strengthens your resolve to continue your intermittent fasting experience.

It's also very important to practice self-compassion. Just as Rome wasn't built in a day, so too are new habits not formed quickly. Recognize that it takes time to get used to intermittent fasting. Instead of seeing setbacks or days when your goals aren't achieved as failures, see them as opportunities for learning. Make adjustments and proceed with optimism.

In conclusion, developing a sustainable and flexible strategy that suits your unique circumstances is the key to setting realistic goals for intermittent fasting. Recognize that every little step counts for your overall well-being and approach it with a positive outlook toward yourself.

Building a Sustainable Routine

In the context of intermittent fasting (IF), developing a sustainable routine is more about designing a lifestyle that suits your individual requirements and preferences than it is about adhering to strict restrictions or deprivation. Together, we will create an IF regimen that is easy to maintain and fits into your everyday schedule.

First, think about your responsibilities and daily schedule. Adjust your fasting window to coincide with your day's natural progression. If you're an early riser, it might be more appropriate for you to begin your fast in the evening. On the other hand, night owls might favor delaying breakfast until later in the day. Making IF work for you rather than the other way around is crucial.

The foundation of intermittent fasting sustainability is meal planning. Accept nutrient-dense foods that will satisfy your hunger and fuel your body when you're fasting. Pay attention to a well-balanced intake of carbohydrates, healthy fats, and proteins. Try different recipes to make your meals interesting, prevent boredom, and develop a healthy relationship with the food you eat.

Maintaining your IF regimen requires staying hydrated. Throughout the day, sip on lots of water to prevent dehydration and control your appetite. Black coffee and herbal teas are also acceptable during the fasting period, offering a tasty respite without interfering with your fasting objectives.

The urge to overeat during times when you're not fasting is one of the traps that many people fall into. Recall that observing intermittent fasting does not give you permission to overindulge in calories. Eat in moderation, enjoy every bite, and develop an awareness of your body's signals of hunger and fullness. By cultivating a more positive relationship with food, this mindful approach helps your IF habit last longer.

Exercise should be a part of any fasting regimen, but it should be customized to your tastes and degree of fitness. Find what makes you happy and content, whether it's an evening workout at the gym, a morning yoga class, or a stroll in the afternoon. Incorporating exercise into intermittent fasting (IF) amplifies its advantages and promotes general health.

During the time you are fasting, pay attention to your body's cues. Do not be afraid to change your fasting window or meal schedule if you feel tired or uncomfortable. There isn't one intermittent fasting strategy that works for everyone; the secret is to be flexible. It's about figuring out the balance that suits you personally.

Meals are a major topic of conversation in social settings, therefore managing this element is essential to the long-term success of an IF regimen. Tell your loved ones about the eating window you have selected so they can help you achieve your objectives. Make sure your social life doesn't become a cause of stress by scheduling your social activities around your fasting hours.

Finally, acknowledge and enjoy your small victories. Celebrate your accomplishments, whether they be milestones in your fasting journey or improvements in your overall health. Developing a sustainable IF routine is a journey of self-care and self-discovery, and celebrating your victories helps you stay consistent with the healthy routines you're forming.

Monitoring Progress and Adjustments

No matter how tiny your victory may be, acknowledge it. Acknowledging your accomplishments, whether they be maintaining your fasting window, selecting nutrient-dense foods, or experiencing an increase in energy, helps you stay motivated. To document your experiences and track shifts in your energy, mood, and general well-being, keep a journal.

It's critical to pay attention to your body at every stage. Keep an eye out for indicators of hunger, changes in energy, and any indications of discomfort. It may be time to reevaluate your fasting strategy if you start to struggle or feel worn out. To better meet your unique demands, think about changing the length, kind, or window of your fast.

Consulting with medical professionals on a regular basis can give you important information about how IF is affecting your health. Keep an eye on important metrics like blood pressure, cholesterol, and blood sugar to make sure they support your wellness objectives. Getting advice from a dietitian or nutritionist can also help you customize your fasting schedule to meet particular dietary requirements.

Recall that the foundation of long-lasting transformation is flexibility. Your attitude to IF should be dynamic, just like life itself. Be willing to modify a specific fasting regimen if unanticipated events or changes in lifestyle make it difficult. Making a strategy that works with your schedule and supports your physical and mental health is the aim.

When it comes to intermittent fasting, progress is more than just physical changes—it's about developing a healthy connection between your body and food. Accept the process of learning, pay attention to your needs, and enjoy the self-discovery journey that results from a continuous commitment to your wellbeing.

CHAPTER 6: Nutrition and Meal Planning

Balancing Macronutrients

In the dynamic realm of intermittent fasting (IF), attaining a balanced and harmonious intake of macronutrients serves as your guide to a successful and healthy journey. Think of it as a symphony in which different parts are played by proteins, lipids, and carbs, all of which contribute to your body's general health.

Let's begin with protein, the main attraction. Proteins, which are sometimes referred to as the "building blocks of life," help your body retain muscular growth, boost immunity, and sustain high energy levels. Maintaining a sufficient protein intake becomes even more important when IF is used. Excellent protein partners on your IF route include lean meats, chicken, fish, eggs, and plant-based sources like beans and lentils. They satisfy your appetite and supply the vital amino acids your body needs to heal and grow.

Let's now add the fat melody. Despite the common belief that fats are bad for you, they are actually essential for a well-rounded IF strategy. Nutrient-dense foods like avocados, nuts, seeds, and olive oil are rich in healthy fats that are essential for hormone balance, brain function, and the absorption of fat-soluble vitamins.

These fats provide a stable beat that grounds your IF experience and improves the nutritional value of your meals as a whole.

And now for the carbohydrates, the steady rhythms that give your IF regimen life. Carbs are a necessary source of energy, even though some diets may demonize them—especially for people who practice intermittent fasting. If you want to consume complex carbohydrates throughout your fasting times, choose whole grains, fruits, and vegetables. These carbohydrates serve as the foundation, giving your body the energy it requires for continuous endurance and vigor.

Let's now discuss how to incorporate these macronutrients into your regular meals. Consider choosing an eating window that fits your lifestyle when you start your IF adventure. Maybe you like a later meal in the evening, or maybe you're an early riser who loves breakfast. Regardless of your inclination, be careful to split up your macronutrient intake throughout the course of your selected eating window.

Eat a high-protein meal to break your fast, such as yogurt, eggs, or protein smoothies, which will boost your metabolism and keep you full. As a mid-morning snack, try avocado on whole-grain toast or a handful of nuts to introduce healthy fats. Add more complex carbs to your main meals throughout the day, such as quinoa, sweet potatoes, or a rainbow of bright veggies. The secret is to strike a balance such that the proteins, fats, and carbohydrates on your plate are all delicious.

Snacking when you should be eating? For a well-rounded energy boost, choose nutrient-dense foods like trail mix that has all three macronutrients, carrot sticks with hummus, or Greek yogurt with berries.

It's critical to pay attention to the distinct rhythm of your body. Try varying the macronutrient combinations you use, and observe the effects on your body. Recall that achieving a satisfying and long-lasting balance that promotes your general well-being is the aim, not perfection.

The harmony of macronutrients is your symphony in the world of intermittent fasting, where time-restricted eating is the tune. Accept the variety of fats, proteins, and carbohydrates, and allow your meals to be a pleasant symphony that powers your IF journey while nourishing your body.

Nutrient-Dense Foods

For those who choose to follow this health-conscious lifestyle, nutrient-dense meals play a vital role in the colorful tapestry of intermittent fasting (IF). It's practically a nutritional dance. Imagine it as a well-balanced, harmonious symphony, with each bite adding to the complex harmony required for maximum health, particularly for women over 50.

A successful IF journey starts with having a solid understanding of nutrient-dense meals and how they affect your body. These foods are necessary for maintaining energy levels, supporting metabolic processes, and boosting general health since they are high in vitamins, minerals, and other essential nutrients.

When it comes to nutrient richness, leafy greens are the main event. In addition to adding a pop of color to your dish, spinach, kale, and Swiss chard are packed full of calcium, iron, and vitamins A, C, and K. These leafy green powerhouses support a sensation of vitality during fasting periods in addition to providing your body with nourishment.

Vegetables come in a wider range of colors than just greens. Bright bell peppers, tomatoes, and carrots provide a powerful antioxidant symphony that fortifies your body's resistance to oxidative stress. In addition to being tasty, these nutrient-dense vegetables give your meals a range of textures and flavors, which will satisfy your palate during the fast.

Lean protein options such as fish, poultry, and tofu are the best. Omega-3 fatty acids, which promote heart health and cognitive function, are especially abundant in salmon and deserve a standing ovation. Conversely, tofu and poultry provide vital amino acids that are necessary for maintaining muscle mass, which is important for women over 50 who want to maintain their lean body mass.

An essential component of the nutrient-dense story is embracing healthy fats. In addition to adding a hint of creamy richness to your meals, avocados, almonds, and olive oil contain monounsaturated fats, which are heart-healthy. These healthy fats not only make your food taste better, but they also help you feel fuller for longer, which makes fasting easier.

Whole grains, like brown rice and quinoa, are the foundation of nutrient-dense carbohydrates. These grains, which are rich in fiber, vitamins, and minerals, provide a steady supply of energy, avoiding the dreaded dips in energy that are sometimes linked to fasting. They help you stick to your chosen IF schedule by promoting a feeling of fullness.

Amidst the great array of foods high in nutrients, don't overlook the significance of dairy or dairy substitutes. For example, Greek yogurt provides both protein and probiotics. In addition to promoting digestive health, these also help provide a sense of fullness and contentment, which is essential for a good IF experience.

Nutrient-dense foods are deserving of the focus in the great performance of intermittent fasting. Recall that eating items that promote your general health and wellbeing is equally as important as abstaining. Thus, let this nutrient-dense, dance-like nutritional feast serve as the beat for your IF lifestyle, guaranteeing a continuous, vibrant, and healthy woman over 50.

Hydration and Supplements

Making wise supplement selections and maintaining enough hydration are essential components of a successful intermittent fasting (IF) experience for women over 50. To make sure you can easily manage this part of your health, let's explore the oceans of supplements and enter the welcoming waters of hydration.

Hydration: Feeding the Oasis of Your Body

Imagine your body as an oasis in the desert, fed only by water, the source of life. Taking care of this oasis is analogous to maintaining appropriate hydration levels during intermittent fasting. When fasting for predetermined lengths of time, it's simple to forget how important it is to stay hydrated.

When a woman over 50 begins intermittent fasting (IF), her body experiences certain changes, making it even more important to stay properly hydrated. Water facilitates the absorption of nutrients, aids in digestion, and keeps the body's fluid balance in a healthy range. It is the unsung hero that works silently to maintain your metabolism.

Throughout your fasting hours, make water your constant buddy. Here's some helpful advice. For a refreshing twist, add a sprig of mint or a splash of citrus. Recall that taking a steady sip might help prevent unneeded hunger pangs and maintain your energy levels.

Supplements: Increasing the Strength of Your Nutrition

Let's embark on our journey into the realm of supplements now. Even while there are many advantages to intermittent fasting, you still need to make sure you're obtaining enough nutrition. Selecting the appropriate supplements can ensure a smooth sail by serving as your co-captains on this adventure.

Support for Vitamins and Minerals: Women over 50 frequently need extra help with specific vitamins and minerals. To strengthen your nutritional base, think about taking supplements like calcium, vitamin D, and B vitamins. These can improve energy levels, promote bone health, and enhance general wellbeing.

Electrolytes: Electrolyte imbalances brought on by fasting can occasionally impair hydration and muscular performance. Including an electrolyte supplement can assist sustain that delicate balance, particularly if you fast for extended periods of time. It's similar to giving your body a tiny treasure trove of nutrients.

Omega-3 Fatty Acids: These good fats can help you reach your best health by acting as the wind in your sails. Supplements containing omega-3 fatty acids promote heart health, improve brain function, and may reduce inflammation. These benefits can be especially helpful for women over 50.

Adaptogens: Your body uses adaptogens as navigators to adjust to stress and changes. Supplements that strengthen your body's resilience and have a relaxing effect, such as rhodiola or ashwagandha, can be helpful during intermittent fasting.

Speak with your healthcare provider before going on a supplement binge. They can offer you advice based on your particular health requirements, making sure the supplements you choose fit your particular profile.

Remember, in this delightful investigation of vitamins and water during intermittent fasting, that the goal should be thriving rather than merely surviving. You're not just surviving the storm; you're charting a course for a healthier, more energetic version of yourself when you feed your body with water and strategically chosen vitamins.

Creating Delicious and Nutritious Meal

Taking up intermittent fasting is an interesting journey that doesn't have to compromise on taste or nutrition. Actually, it opens up a world of tasty and nourishing meals that can improve your health and add enjoyment to your fasting periods.

Imagine a meal that is bursting with taste, color, and nutrients that are specifically designed to support your body during periods of intermittent fasting. Let's explore the art of preparing meals that will satisfy your body and provide it with all the nourishment it needs.

Eat a meal that will nourish your body and taste buds to start the day off well. Imagine a thick omelet topped with tomatoes, feta cheese, and lush greens. Your metabolism will be accelerated and your energy levels sustained throughout the morning with the combination of protein and vital vitamins.

Enjoy a nutrient-dense salad for lunch that consists of a mix of vibrant vegetables, lean protein (such chickpeas or grilled chicken), and a sprinkle of olive oil. This light dinner will satisfy your hunger and supply your body with the vital nutrition it requires.

Enjoy a filling dinner of lean protein, healthy fats, and whole grains as your intermittent fasting eating window draws near. Suggest a baked salmon filet accompanied by roasted veggies and quinoa. Salmon's omega-3 fatty acids support heart health, and quinoa offers a nutritious source of energy.

You can enjoy snacking as a part of your fasting regimen. Choose a handful of nuts or seeds, such as chia or almond seeds, to add a healthy fat boost and a satisfying crunch. For a satisfying and well-rounded snack, combine them with some fruit.

Staying hydrated is essential. To add a refreshing touch, add cucumber, mint, or citrus fruit slices to your water. Herbal teas provide warmth and flavor without adding extra calories, making them excellent fasting companions as well.

Try varying the herbs and spices in your cooking to improve the flavor without using a lot of sauce or seasoning. A basic meal can be elevated to a culinary masterpiece with the correct combination, adding to the pleasure of your intermittent fasting.

Never forget that balance and diversity are essential for successful intermittent fasting. In addition to meeting your body's nutritional demands, you may make your fasting times exciting by embracing a wide variety of tasty and nourishing meals. Thus, when you embark on your intermittent fasting adventure, let your taste buds rejoice as you enjoy the goodness of carefully prepared, nourishing meals.

CHAPTER 7: Managing Hunger and Cravings

Strategies for Overcoming Hunger

A straightforward tactic that is often disregarded is maintaining adequate hydration. Our bodies frequently mistake thirst for hunger. Therefore, consider drinking some water, herbal tea, or black coffee before reaching for food. These drinks can help you feel full and reduce appetite in addition to providing you with necessary hydration.

Arrange Your Meals Well

Creating meals that are nutrient-dense and well-balanced is essential to controlling hunger when fasting intermittently. To provide you long-lasting energy, make sure your meals contain a variety of proteins, good fats, and complex carbohydrates. Remember that foods high in fiber, such as fruits, vegetables, and whole grains, help with digestion and promote a sensation of fullness.

Plan Your Meal Times Wisely

Think about timing your meals to coincide with your fasting windows. Arrange your meals to fit within your eating window if you're adhering to an intermittent fasting regimen. By teaching your body to expect nourishment during those certain times, this can help control hunger and make the fasting hours more tolerable.

Optimum Nutrition Consumption

Persistent hunger might occasionally be an indication that your body lacks certain nutrients. Verify that you're getting enough vitamins and minerals because insufficient amounts can make you feel hungry. Examine nutrient-dense foods and seek advice from a nutritionist if necessary to make sure your dietary decisions are promoting your general well-being.

Pay Attention to Your Body

It's critical to recognize the indications of hunger produced by your body. During your eating window, respect your genuine hunger. The goal of intermittent fasting is to establish a sustainable rhythm rather than to deprive yourself. Forging a positive relationship with food can be achieved by being aware of your hunger cues, eating thoughtfully, and enjoying your food.

Add Satisfying Foods

Make an effort to include foods that are naturally satiety-promoting. Lean meats, beans, and dairy products are high in protein and can help you feel fuller for longer. Healthy fats from nuts, avocados, and olive oil are good sources of fat and also help to make you feel satisfied. Try a variety of foods to find what sustains your sense of nourishment during your fasting intervals.

Continue to be preoccupied and distracted.

Keeping your thoughts occupied might be an effective strategy to combat hunger. Plan your activities, complete assignments, or engage in hobbies while you're fasting. This serves to both divert your attention from your hunger and establish a favorable relationship with your fasting intervals.

Modify Your Fasting Window Gradually

If you are still hungry, you might choose to progressively extend your window for fasting. Start with a shorter fasting period and progressively lengthen it over time rather than diving into a lengthy one. This makes it easier for your body to adjust to the new food routine.

Control Your Stress Levels

Emotional eating brought on by stress can interfere with your fasting experience. Include stress-relieving practices in your regimen, such as yoga, meditation, or deep breathing exercises. During intermittent fasting, these behaviors boost your general well-being in addition to helping you manage stress.

To sum up, managing hunger while on an intermittent fast entails a blend of deliberate eating, tactical planning, and being aware of your body's cues. You'll improve your experience with intermittent fasting overall and be able to manage hunger more skillfully if you include these helpful tactics into your daily routine. Recall that the goal is to strike a balance that supports both a long-term and pleasurable fasting experience for you.

Dealing with Cravings

For women over fifty, starting an intermittent fasting journey can be empowering and transforming, but let's face it—there are drawbacks as well. Chief among these are persistent cravings that seem to nag at the most inconvenient moments. Do not be alarmed! It takes more than just resolve to overcome cravings; instead, you must understand your body and develop coping mechanisms that will make the process joyful and long-lasting.

Understanding the Source of Cravings

It's important to remember that cravings are your body's friendly cues that something particular is needed. Try interpreting the signals your appetites are trying to convey rather than giving in to or opposing them. Frequently, they may indicate that your body is deficient in specific nutrients or that you are actually thirsty instead of hungry. It all comes down to observing the minute cues.

Maintain Hydration and Pay Attention to Your Body

Staying well hydrated is one of the easiest yet most effective strategies to reduce cravings. Sometimes, urges or hunger are just disguises for dehydration. Make it a habit to drink water when you're fasting. Try different herbal teas or infused water to keep things interesting and satisfy your palate without breaking your fast.

Eating Consciously During Feeding Times

When it comes time to break your fast, commit to eating mindfully. Take a seat, enjoy every meal, and focus on the tastes and textures. Using all of your senses when eating not only makes the meal more enjoyable overall but also makes it easier for your brain to recognize fullness, which lowers the risk of giving in to cravings after the meal.

Modified Nutrient Consumption

Make sure each of your meals has a good balance of complex carbohydrates, healthy fats, and proteins. In addition to offering lasting energy, a balanced plate reduces the likelihood of feeling deprived, which can lead to cravings. Try incorporating visually appealing and nutritious foods into your meals by experimenting with bright, nutrient-dense items.

Clever Snacking Techniques

The concept of nibbling while on an intermittent fast may seem paradoxical to many people. Snacking with purpose and awareness, however, can be a very effective strategy to combat cravings. To stay full, choose high-fiber and high-protein snacks. Healthy options such as nuts, seeds, Greek yogurt, or sliced veggies with hummus won't interfere with your fasting objectives.

Enjoy yourself Sensibly, Not irrationally

Sometimes, cravings make you want for particular foods, and depriving yourself completely could backfire. Sometimes you should treat yourself, but only when you are conscious and inside your mealtime window. Enjoy a modest portion of your favorite dessert or a piece of dark chocolate without feeling guilty. Recall that sustainability over the long term and balance are key.

Stress Reduction and Self-Taking

Stress levels often cause cravings to resurface. Include stress-reduction strategies in your daily routine, such as deep breathing, meditation, or a relaxing pastime. A key component of a fruitful intermittent fasting journey is taking good care of your mental and emotional health.

Essentially, managing cravings during intermittent fasting is a dance that involves being aware of and attentive to your body's signals rather than a fight. Accept the process, pay attention to your body, and see every urge as a chance to discover more about yourself on this enjoyable and rewarding path to a better, healthier version of yourself.

Psychological Aspects of Fasting

Let's start by talking about the mentality shift that comes with intermittent fasting. Rewiring your relationship with food and accepting a new approach to sustaining your body is more important than simply skipping meals. Women typically have to mentally adapt as they get older to meet the changing needs of their bodies. We are invited to see food as fuel for vitality rather than just a regular need when we observe intermittent fasting.

Empowerment is one of the main psychological advantages of IF. When they actively choose when to eat, many women over 50 experience a restored sense of control over their health and well-being. This independence can provide self-assurance and a positive outlook, which can help one feel accomplished for sticking to a fasting schedule.

Additionally, intermittent fasting promotes conscious eating. It naturally encourages a greater awareness of hunger and satiety cues with mealtime windows. This increased consciousness can result in a more purposeful and joyful connection with food. Women might find themselves enjoying every piece of food rather than just scarfing it down, which would improve the entire eating experience.

Any change in lifestyle, including intermittent fasting, might present difficulties. Women over 50 who are used to traditional eating patterns could find it difficult to adjust to a new regimen. It's critical to face these difficulties with optimism. Acknowledge that mistakes may occasionally happen and treat them as learning experiences and opportunities to improve rather than as setbacks.

Self-discovery is one of IF's main psychological features. Women may discover emotional ties to food and long-standing behaviors as they investigate this novel eating strategy. Being self-aware can help you make well-informed decisions about your diet and general health.

The perspective of time is also affected by intermittent fasting. The set eating windows can assist women over 50 better manage their daily routines by establishing a sense of rhythm and habit. Their lives will feel more balanced and less stressful as a result of their increased structure.

The resilience that intermittent fasting cultivates is another aspect of its psychological effects. Women who become accustomed to fasting cycles frequently find an inner power they were unaware they had. Beyond the domain of eating habits, mental toughness and resilience can be developed by overcoming hunger sensations and restraining the impulse to eat outside of set hours.

Intermittent fasting can also change how people interact when they eat. Women could discover that they need to reconsider the social relationships they have when it comes to food. This change doesn't imply giving up on fun dinners with loved ones; rather, it means adjusting and coming up with new ideas for connecting without depending entirely on customary mealtimes.

In summary, the psychological benefits of intermittent fasting for women over 50 surpass the physiological modifications. It's about developing an empowered mindset, rediscovering a fresh relationship with food, and accepting a positive outlook. Intermittent fasting can evolve beyond a food preference to a holistic approach to wellbeing that benefits the mind, body, and spirit via mindfulness, resilience, and self-discovery. Thus, when you begin your adventure of intermittent fasting, keep in mind that taking care of your mind and spirit is just as important as what you eat.

Building a Healthy Relationship with Food

When it comes to intermittent fasting, developing a positive relationship with food transcends beyond diet and becomes a way of life that satisfies the body and the mind. Let's take a trip that goes beyond simple nourishment and concentrates on the crucial element of developing a healthy and harmonious relationship with the food you eat.

Understanding Hunger as a Guide:

The increased awareness of hunger cues that comes with intermittent fasting is one of the most amazing changes. Consider hunger as a helpful guide rather than as an enemy. Pay attention to the cues your body gives you and use them as a guide. An awareness of your body's requirements is fostered by intuitive eating, which is a practice entwined with intermittent fasting that teaches you to respect your natural pattern of hunger and fullness.

Breaking Free from Emotional Eating:

Releasing food from emotional triggers is a necessary step in developing a positive connection with it. You can recognize emotional eating behaviors by using the reflective space that intermittent fasting provides. Consider for a moment if you're eating to satiate true hunger or whether you're eating to cope with stress, boredom, or other feelings. Understanding and resolving your emotional attachment to food gives you the ability to make deliberate decisions.

Enjoying Each Bite:

Meals frequently turn into hurried affairs due to the bustle of daily life. A period of intermittent fasting encourages you to take things slowly and mindfully enjoy every meal. Accept and enjoy the tastes, scents, and textures of food as a sensory experience. You can build gratitude for the nourishment that comes from eating by being fully present throughout meals, which also enhances the enjoyment of the food itself.

Cultivating a Diverse Plate:

Variety is the flavor of life, and this also applies to the foods you choose to eat. A varied and well-balanced approach to eating is promoted by intermittent fasting. To guarantee a wide range of nutrients, try a rainbow of fruits, veggies, whole grains, and lean meats. Including variety in your diet improves general health and adds to a more pleasurable and fulfilling dining experience.

Closing Nutritional Divides:

It is not necessary to forgo important nutrients when fasting intermittently. During eating windows, concentrate on consuming nutrient-dense foods that will best nourish your body. Include a variety of minerals, vitamins, and antioxidants to promote general health. Consciously attending to your nutritional demands cultivates a sense of accountability for your overall well-being.

Mindfully Honoring Indulgences:

Balance is key to a healthy relationship with food rather than rigid regulations. Flexibility is made possible by intermittent fasting, including the odd indulgence. It's important to handle these situations with balance and attention. Treats should be enjoyed guilt-free, enjoyed as a part of life's pleasures rather than giving in to cycles of binge eating.

The road to developing a positive connection with food is a dynamic and unique experience when it comes to intermittent fasting. It entails introspection, making deliberate decisions, and celebrating the positive relationship that exists between what you eat and your general health. So, relish every bite, pay attention to your body, and allow your body to lead you to a balanced and pleasurable relationship with food through intermittent fasting.

CHAPTER 8: Exercise and Physical Activity

Incorporating Exercise into Fasting

The deliberate integration of exercise into your fasting regimen is a crucial component that amplifies these advantages. Incorporating physical exercise into your fasting window enhances the benefits on your metabolism and enhances your general health.

Let's examine how adding exercise to your intermittent fasting regimen can be a happy and fulfilling decision. It's crucial to select exercises based on your fitness level and personal preferences first and foremost. Whether it's weight training, mild yoga, or brisk walking, selecting an exercise that you enjoy can keep you motivated and assure sustainability.

Intermittent fasting combined with exercise can help boost fat burning. Physical activity enhances the method by which your body uses stored energy during fasting to support effective weight management. Fasting and exercise work in unison to generate a harmonious rhythm that is beneficial to your overall health, much like in a dance.

Exercise during a fast can also improve insulin sensitivity, which is important for people dealing with the effects of aging. Your body uses glucose more efficiently when insulin sensitivity is higher, which lowers the risk of insulin resistance and type 2 diabetes. It's similar to giving your metabolic system a revitalizing tune-up that enables it to perform at its best.

Maintaining bone density becomes more important for women over 50. It might be likened to weaving a strong and resilient skeleton by including weight-bearing workouts into your fasting time. This helps to avoid osteoporosis, which is a significant worry as we age, in addition to supporting bone health. Think of it as strengthening the base of your body and guaranteeing durability for many years to come.

Exercise during intermittent fasting provides tremendous benefits for mental health in addition to physical health. Endorphins, also known as the "feel-good" chemicals, are released while you are under stress and can improve your mood. It's like taking your thoughts on a rejuvenating journey, resulting in an upbeat and joyful experience.

For women over 50, combining exercise and intermittent fasting is essentially a celebration of your body's resiliency and strength rather than just a regimen. It's about developing a way of life that supports emotional and physical well-being. Put on your sneakers, spread out your yoga mat, and savor the energizing combination of exercise and fasting. Your lively symphony will be appreciated by your body, mind, and soul.

Tailoring Workouts to Age and Fitness Level

It's critical to adjust your routines based on your age and degree of fitness. The good news is that exercise can support your intermittent fasting regimen and enhance general health and vigor if done properly.

First, let's talk about the age component. Changes in bone density, hormone balance, and muscle mass are common in women over 50. Selecting workouts that address these particular demands is crucial. You should think about adding resistance training to your exercise routine. Resistance bands, free weights, and bodyweight exercises can all help achieve this. Strength exercise promotes bone health, which is more crucial as we age, in addition to helping to maintain and grow muscle.

Exercises that target the heart are another essential element. Swimming, cycling, and brisk walking are exercises that increase heart health and endurance. It's critical to adjust the intensity of these exercises to your current level of fitness. Set out at a speed that will test you but still permit steady improvement. Recall that the goal should be consistency and long-term gains rather than going above and beyond.

Exercises for balance and flexibility are often neglected, yet as we age, they become increasingly important. Include exercises like tai chi or yoga in your schedule. These improve balance and coordination in addition to increasing flexibility. Preventing falls and preserving joint mobility are essential components of total fitness as we age.

Let's now talk about how important it is to modify your workouts based on your current level of fitness. Regardless of your level of experience, finding a balance that pushes you without putting you under too much stress is essential. Pay attention to your body's signals and move at a comfortable speed.

If you've never exercised before, start with low-impact exercises like light yoga or walking. As your body adjusts, progressively up the intensity and time. If you already have a fitness regimen, think about incorporating interval training or higher-intensity exercises, just make sure they fit in with your fasting schedule.

Particularly advantageous is interval training, which switches between brief bursts of high-intensity activity and rest or lower-intensity intervals. It not only improves cardiovascular health but also enhances the metabolic advantages of intermittent fasting. This strategy supports your overall health goals by burning calories both during and after your workout.

Keeping your workouts varied is essential to avoiding boredom and maintaining enthusiasm. To keep things interesting, experiment with various hobbies. This could entail a weekly regimen that combines strength, cardio, and flexibility training. Try out a variety of workouts to find what you enjoy the most so that you can look forward to your fitness regimen.

Never forget that every fitness regimen must include both rest and recovery. Sufficient rest, appropriate hydration, and letting your body heal in between workouts all help you perform at your best and lower your chance of injury.

To sum up, adjusting your exercise regimen to your age and level of fitness is a smart move that will guarantee a pleasurable and successful intermittent fasting experience. Accept the variety of workouts, put consistency before intensity, and acknowledge your progress as you go. Treat your body with respect and it will reward you with more energy, strength, and vitality. Your body is a special and robust vessel.

Benefits of Combining Exercise with Intermittent Fasting

Exercise combined with intermittent fasting becomes a potent combination in the colorful tapestry of life, particularly for women in their golden years. Together, they not only help the body become healthier but also set off a series of advantages that improve mental and physical health.

Imagine this: when you exercise consistently throughout your fasting window, your body turns like a metabolic maestro, arranging favorable alterations in a symphony. The increased burning of fat is one of the main factors in this performance. Your body becomes an expert fat-burning machine when you workout while fasting because it can access its fat stores more quickly. This helps to maintain a leaner, more toned body in addition to helping with weight management.

Exercising combined with intermittent fasting ignites a metabolic firestorm, regardless of appearances. Growth hormone is produced at a rate that explodes in your body, promoting the growth and repair of muscle. This is particularly important for women over 50 because it helps prevent the aging-related natural loss of muscle mass. In addition to supporting bodily functions, stronger muscles increase metabolism, which facilitates maintaining a healthy weight.

The mutually reinforcing advantages penetrate the cognitive as well as the physical domains. Regular activity creates an abundance of endorphins, which are happy hormones that can lighten even the most difficult fasting hours. Intermittent fasting combined with physical activity has also been connected to better brain health and cognitive performance. It gives your mind a double dose of vigor.

Let's now discuss the wonders of insulin sensitivity. Your body responds more favorably to insulin, the hormone in charge of controlling blood sugar, when you exercise while fasting sometimes. This increased sensitivity lowers the likelihood of type 2 diabetes and insulin resistance, which is revolutionary. This becomes a useful defense against age-related health issues for women over 50, whose bodies may naturally become less sensitive to insulin.

Consider your body to be a sturdy ship traveling through time. Combining intermittent fasting with exercise serves as a compass that points your vessel in the direction of better cardiovascular health. By lowering blood pressure, cholesterol, and improving overall cardiovascular function, the pair promotes heart health. It's similar to giving your heart a daily hug and kiss.

Not to mention the energy boost that results from this well-balanced mix. Despite popular belief, exercise during intermittent fasting promotes higher energy levels rather than weariness. You'll experience an increase in energy and alertness throughout the day as your body gets better at using the stored energy, making every moment of the day seem like an adventure.

Exercise combined with intermittent fasting is a melody of well-being in the big symphony of life. It's about adopting a lifestyle that supports your body, mind, and spirit—it's not just about losing weight or building muscle. So, for a healthier, happier you, lace up those shoes, enjoy the joy of movement, and let the intermittent fasting melody blend harmoniously with the beat of exercise.

CHAPTER 9: Potential Health Concerns and Precautions

Consultation with Healthcare Professionals

Adopting any lifestyle change requires open and honest conversation with healthcare providers, and intermittent fasting for women over 50 is no exception. This consultation provides an invaluable starting point for a safe, customized fasting experience based on each person's unique health requirements.

Talking to your healthcare practitioner at the outset of your intermittent fasting adventure is like having an informed ally at your side. This collaborative approach guarantees consideration of any pre-existing health issues, prescriptions, or concerns. Your healthcare provider is well-versed in your medical background and may provide advice tailored to your particular health profile.

Being truthful is essential when talking to your healthcare practitioner about intermittent fasting. Tell us about your reasons for wanting to lose weight, improve your energy, or just feel better overall. This information assists your healthcare provider in giving you advice that takes your health condition into account and is in line with your goals.

A crucial component of the session is answering any worries or inquiries you might have regarding intermittent fasting. Your doctor can provide further information about the potential effects of fasting on blood pressure, blood sugar, and cholesterol. It's essential to comprehend these possible consequences in order to make wise choices regarding your fasting schedule.

Furthermore, based on your medical history, healthcare specialists can assist in identifying any warning signs or prospective problems. For instance, people with diabetes, heart problems, or specific hormone imbalances might need a more customized approach to intermittent fasting. Working together with your healthcare practitioner will guarantee that your fasting strategy is safe, sustainable, and successful.

It's critical to see this consultation as a continuous dialogue. It's important to update your healthcare practitioner about your experiences with intermittent fasting and any changes you notice in your health as you go along. This conversation enables you to modify your fasting regimen so that it continues to be beneficial to your overall health.

It is crucial to talk about when to take drugs during fasting times for people who could be taking them.

Medical specialists can provide advice on how to keep your medication regimen effective by coordinating your fasting pattern with it.

Your healthcare provider can provide holistic assistance by taking into account the psychological and emotional effects of fasting in addition to medical ones. They can offer you advice on how to implement intermittent fasting while also regulating your stress levels, sleep schedule, and general mental health.

Recall that your healthcare practitioner exists to help and empower you. Be open-minded and prepared to work together to create a strategy that supports your health objectives when you go into the session. Because of this connection, you can feel secure and confident that you are starting your intermittent fasting journey under the direction of a reliable healthcare provider.

Essentially, one of the most important steps in appropriately incorporating intermittent fasting into your life is to speak with healthcare professionals. It's a conversation that prioritizes your health, making sure that fasting is not only successful but also improves your general state of health.

Addressing Pre-existing Conditions

Starting an intermittent fast can be a thrilling adventure that leads to health and regeneration. To guarantee a safe and customized approach to this lifestyle shift, there may be some extra considerations for people with pre-existing conditions.

Firstly and foremost, before embarking on the intermittent fasting seas, it is imperative that you speak with your healthcare provider. With their knowledgeable compass, your doctor can help you navigate any obstacles and create a plan that is in line with your medical requirements. By taking this step, you can make sure that your fasting strategy is both easy on your body and effective.

It becomes especially important to consider the time and type of fasting periods for people who are managing diseases such as diabetes or cardiovascular difficulties. Blood sugar levels can be affected by intermittent fasting, thus people with diabetes need to be extremely careful. Work together with your medical team to come up with a fasting plan that won't affect the stability of your blood sugar.

Intermittent fasting can be beneficial or detrimental to heart health. On the one hand, it might help with better metabolic markers and weight loss, both of which are good for heart health. Conversely, the stress associated with fasting may affect blood pressure. If you're experiencing heart-related issues, your physician can assist you in finding the best balance and track your development.

Many people struggle with thyroid problems, which calls for a more sophisticated approach to intermittent fasting. Abrupt alterations in dietary habits may impact thyroid function. Your doctor can create a customized strategy that takes into account your thyroid's requirements so that you can benefit from fasting without disturbing this delicate balance.

Particular attention may be needed for digestive problems including irritable bowel syndrome (IBS) or inflammatory bowel illnesses. It's important to collaborate with your healthcare team to create a strategy that takes your gut health into account, as intermittent fasting may exacerbate symptoms.

A caring approach is necessary when implementing intermittent fasting for people who have a history of eating disorders. Sometimes fasting sets off harmful habits or ways of thinking. Work together with a medical expert who specializes in managing eating disorders to create a strategy that promotes a healthy relationship with food.

The physiological stress of fasting can increase chronic stress, a silent companion for many. Prioritizing stress-reduction strategies like mindfulness, meditation, or light exercise is essential. Recall that intermittent fasting should improve your general wellbeing rather than cause you more stress.

Pay close attention to your body's cues as you go on your intermittent fast. Pay attention to the signals it gives, and be honest with your healthcare team if you have any worries or unusual reactions. You can make changes to your plan to guarantee a safe and easy travel.

The route to wellbeing is via a customized, all-encompassing approach. Your individual navigational map that leads you to the best possible health includes your pre-existing illnesses. You can customize your intermittent fasting experience and turn it into a journey of self-discovery and well-being by working with your healthcare providers.

Monitoring and Adjusting for Optimal Health

Recognizing that each person is unique and that what works for one may not work for another is crucial. As we begin our investigation into intermittent fasting, see it as a customized experience based on your unique requirements and health objectives.

Following your body's cues is like having a trustworthy compass on this voyage. Keep a close eye on how your body reacts to times when you fast. Do you have energy or are you starting to feel tired? Is your mental clarity getting better or are you still feeling foggy? You can modify your fasting regimen as needed by following these cues.

Consultations with medical professionals on a frequent basis are essential to keeping an eye on your health while on an intermittent fast. This guarantees that you will be accompanied on this adventure by an informed guide who will assist you in navigating any possible health issues. These experts are essential to preserving your health because they may modify fasting techniques to fit your unique health profile or address pre-existing concerns with you.

Our bodies change as we get older, so things that used to operate perfectly might need to be adjusted. Pay attention to the beat of your body and be willing to adjust as necessary. For example, experiment with different fasting techniques or modify the length of the fasting windows. Discovering a sustainable rhythm that supports optimal health and is in line with your body's requirements is the aim.

In this journey, nutrition is crucial. Make sure your diet stays nutrient-dense and balanced by evaluating it on a regular basis. Do you consume enough minerals and vitamins? Are you using a range of complete foods?

During intermittent fasting, you can greatly improve your general health and well-being by modifying your meal plans in light of these factors.

Water is an essential travel companion that cannot be skipped. It is imperative to maintain enough hydration levels. In addition to sustaining biological processes, water also helps to reduce hunger. To stay as hydrated as possible during the day, have a water bottle nearby and take little sips.

Adopting a flexible perspective is yet another crucial component of this investigation. Because life is dynamic, unexpected things might happen. Consider breaks from your fasting regimen as opportunities to grow and adjust rather than as setbacks. Being adaptable increases resilience, which improves the sustainability and enjoyment of your intermittent fasting experience.

When it comes to intermittent fasting, the art of monitoring and modifying is crucial to achieving optimal health. It's a live, breathing approach to wellbeing rather than a strict set of guidelines. You may confidently sail the waters of intermittent fasting by being aware of your body, working with healthcare professionals, and making the necessary adjustments along the way. This will ensure that your health always stays in the North Star that guides your particular trip.

CHAPTER 10: Success Stories and Inspirational Accounts

Real-Life Experiences of Women Over 50

Here is a compilation of true stories that shed light on the amazing experiences of women over 50 who have dabbled in intermittent fasting in order to regain their strength and energy. You'll learn about the various ways these inspiring ladies have adopted the practices of intermittent fasting and transformed their lives as we dig into these first-person narratives.

Introducing Susan, a vibrant 53-year-old who felt the slowing effects of age and made the decision to take control of her health. Susan found comfort in the 16/8 fasting approach, which limits her daily eating window to eight hours. She describes with contagious enthusiasm how this strategy gave her a sense of empowerment over her well-being in addition to igniting her energy levels.

Linda, a grandma in her early sixties, found that sticking to a 5:2 diet was a sustainable means of keeping her weight in check. She talks about how her friends and family were initially skeptical of her intermittent fasting regimen, but in the end, she found freedom in it. On the days she wasn't fasting, Linda enjoyed cooking nutrient-dense meals and enjoying the harmony of her dietary choices.

As she worked through the difficulties of menopause, 56-year-old Carol tried fasting on alternate days. She embraces the beneficial effects on her hormonal balance while openly sharing the highs and lows of adjusting to this strategy. Carol's story shows how women over 50 can develop resilience in order to successfully negotiate the challenging landscape of midlife and beyond.

Karen, who is in her mid-50s, struggled to balance her demanding work and family obligations, which left her with little time for long workouts. Karen embraced the 12/12 approach after becoming intrigued by its simplicity. Her experience demonstrates how well fasting can be incorporated into a busy routine and shows how even minor adjustments can have a big impact on one's health.

It becomes clear as we delve deeper into these stories that the women's reasons for adopting intermittent fasting are just as varied as they are. Whatever her reason for wanting to lose weight, regulate her energy levels, or enhance her general health, every lady discovered a customized strategy that fit her way of life.

These ladies are united by a common goal to redefine aging. Adopting a more deliberate and attentive relationship with food was sparked by intermittent fasting. These ladies have found a newfound sense of purpose in their everyday lives, from appreciating the ease of feeding their bodies to learning the delights of cooking healthful meals.

The psychological and emotional changes are just as significant. Beyond bodily changes, many describe a deeper self-awareness and self-love. They have found a source of strength that goes beyond the surface by accepting the wisdom that comes with age and the beauty of their age through the lens of intermittent fasting.

You will find moments of vulnerability, resiliency, and victory woven throughout their experiences. These ladies exemplify the spirit of a common journey, demonstrating that growing older is not a barrier but rather a blank canvas on which they can continue to create vivid and meaningful lives.

I hope that reading these stories will encourage you with the bravery and perseverance of these women who have faced midlife with dignity and resolve. Their experiences testify to the transforming potential of intermittent fasting, offering women over 50 who want to fully embrace life's second act a ray of hope and possibilities.

Overcoming Challenges

Starting an intermittent fast can be a thrilling and powerful experience, particularly for women over 50 who want to improve their health. However, it has its own set of difficulties, just like any route to wellness. Do not be alarmed; not only is it possible to overcome these obstacles, but doing so can make for an extremely rewarding experience. Together, we will examine the realm of intermittent fasting and how to overcome any challenges that may arise.

Challenge 1: Taming the Hunger Dragon

Yes, the growling stomach is a frequent traveling companion when following a fast. Managing hunger pangs is one of the main obstacles, particularly in the early stages. Don't worry, it's not a legendary dragon—it's doable! To help your body adjust, start by progressively increasing your window for fasting. To stave off hunger, drink herbal teas, stay hydrated, and choose nutrient-dense meals. Accept the way your body is changing, and you'll find the dragon subdued in no time.

Challenge 2: Social Situations and the Feast of Temptation

An unexpected twist to social events where food plays a prominent role can come from intermittent fasting. Although it may appear difficult, navigating through meals and brunches doesn't have to be difficult. Tell your loved ones about the eating window you've selected, and don't be scared to make changes. At feasts, make thoughtful choices and enjoy the food without feeling obligated to try everything. Recall that the company is just as important as the food.

Challenge 3: Fine-Tuning the Fasting Routine

Establishing the perfect fasting schedule takes time and tweaking, just like tuning a musical instrument. The 16/8 technique may work well for some people, while alternate-day fasting may be preferred for others. Pay attention to the rhythm of your body and try out several methods until you find the one that works best for you. Being adaptable is essential because it enables you to modify your fasting schedule as your lifestyle changes.

Challenge 4: The Emotional Rollercoaster

The journey of intermittent fasting is not just physical but also emotional. There will be days when you feel like you're on top of the world and days when you feel doubtful and frustrated. It's critical to accept these feelings without passing judgment. Consult your family, friends, and online networks for support. Accept the process as a necessary component of your own development and remember that obstacles are just stepping stones to achievement.

Challenge 5: Balancing Nutrition and Nourishment

It's important to keep a balanced diet during intermittent fasting, but finding the correct balance can be difficult. Make sure every meal is nutrient-dense by including a range of fruits, vegetables, lean meats, and healthy fats. Try a variety of meals to keep your taste intrigued, and think about speaking with a nutritionist for individualized advice. Keep in mind that proper nutrition for your body involves more than just fasting.

Challenge 6: Plateaus and Patience

One of the most common obstacles to intermittent fasting is reaching weight reduction plateaus. Understanding that progress isn't always linear is essential. Celebrate your non-scale successes, like increased vitality or sharper thinking. Your best ally is patience; allow your body the time it requires to adjust. If needed, modify your strategy, but don't allow brief plateaus to weaken your resolve.

Challenge 7: Listening to Your Body's Symphony

It's important to listen to your body's unique symphony when facing obstacles. Be mindful of your general well-being, energy levels, and hunger cues. Don't be scared to try a different fasting strategy if you find that one isn't working for you. Recall that the goal of this journey is to find what makes you feel your best and to cultivate a harmonious relationship with your body.

In conclusion, women over 50 who choose to follow an intermittent fasting path will find it to be an exhilarating journey with obstacles that deepen the experience. Accept every challenge as a chance for development, education, and self-discovery. You may overcome the obstacles with grace and use them as stepping stones to a happier, healthier version of yourself if you have an optimistic outlook, are adaptable, and have a little humor. Let's toast to overcoming the challenges and relishing the fulfilling experience of sporadic fasting!

Celebrating Achievements

There's a special thread that runs through the colorful fabric of life, telling the stories of innumerable women over 50 who have chosen intermittent fasting (IF). When we explore the celebration of successes in this transforming field, we discover stories of empowerment that go hand in hand with physical changes.

The beauty of acknowledging successes in intermittent fasting is found in the significant influence it has on one's general health as well as the outward changes. Imagine this: as each day of her IF journey goes by, the woman loses weight and gains confidence while simultaneously shedding self-doubt.

The range of experiences in IF success tales is one amazing feature. Meet Susan, a lively woman in her early 50s who started an IF practice and found a fresh feeling of vitality and energy. She smiles and says, "I used to think that being older was a barrier to feeling energetic, but intermittent fasting has completely changed that perspective for me."

For a lot of people, success lies not only in the numbers on a scale but also in being freed from the constraints of continual calorie counting. "I've spent years meticulously counting calories, and with intermittent fasting, it's like a breath of fresh air," says 56-year-old Linda, an IF devotee. It has made a huge difference that it's not just about what I consume, but also when."

Not only are physical changes celebrated, but also mental and emotional breakthroughs. Women are emerging from the cycle of emotional eating, and their capacity to manage their relationship with food provides them with power and comfort. It's a liberation dance, an interior metamorphosis that coexists with the outward shifts.

Jane, a 58-year-old supporter of intermittent fasting, shares her emotional victory: "I learned to listen to my body through intermittent fasting." Not only am I feeding it physically, but I'm feeding it emotionally too. I never would have imagined that a holistic approach could give me such a sense of tranquility and attentiveness."

What's even more touching about IF success tales is their social component. Women build communities, encouraging and supporting one another as they overcome common obstacles and successes. The accomplishment is a group celebration of fortitude and unity as much as an individual triumph.

A prevalent theme among the successes of intermittent fasting is self-discovery. Women realize their inherent strength, which is often eclipsed by cultural expectations. It's a celebration of embracing the strength that comes with experience and knowledge and escaping the confines of age-related stereotypes.

IF develops into a path of self-love, where accomplishments are about accepting and loving one's body at every stage of life rather than just fitting into a specific dress size. The idea is aptly expressed by 53-year-old IF fan Helen, who says, "It's not about looking a certain way; it's about feeling alive and appreciating the vessel that carries me through this beautiful journey of life."

The delight of taking back time is just as much of an accomplishment in intermittent fasting as it is in the physical, emotional, and social domains. Women rejoice in their newfound independence from the demands of meal planning every day and discover that they have more time for the things they want to do.

While we commemorate these successes, let's also recognize that each woman's IF narrative is distinct. It's not a story that works for everyone; rather, it's a symphony of unique stories that all add to the chorus of empowerment and wellbeing. Thus, let's celebrate the successes—both large and tiny, apparent and hidden—that contribute to the genuinely life-changing and fulfilling experience of intermittent fasting for women over 50.

Conclusion

Recap of Key Points

For women over 50, navigating the world of intermittent fasting is like setting out on a quest for improved health and wellbeing. We have discovered a wealth of useful information and insights that can be easily incorporated into your everyday routine as a result of our investigation. Let's take a time to review the essential information that will act as your trustworthy roadmap to a better version of yourself.

First and foremost, a solid foundation is established by comprehending the fundamentals of intermittent fasting. It's a lifestyle change that embraces your body's natural rhythm rather than just a diet. Realizing the significance of this strategy can lead to profound modifications in your hormonal and metabolic balance, especially for women over 50.

Examining the physiology of intermittent fasting in greater detail reveals the complex interplay between your body's systems. The main stage is occupied by metabolism, which adapts in a rhythmic and harmonious manner. The overall efficacy of this approach is attributed to hormonal changes, particularly the favorable influence on insulin sensitivity. Furthermore, autophagy—a mechanism that repairs cells—becomes increasingly important for preserving the health of cells, particularly as we age.

Adapting intermittent fasting to the special requirements of women over fifty turns into an essential part of your journey. Acknowledging and managing hormonal shifts is like fine-tuning your health instrument. This personalization includes taking into account each person's unique lifestyle, dietary needs, and possible obstacles. It's important to create a plan that is in line with your unique requirements and objectives rather than taking a one-size-fits-all approach.

You learn about the variety of alternatives available as you investigate common intermittent fasting techniques, like the 16/8 method, 5:2 diet, alternate-day fasting, and extended fasting. Instead of rigorously following a schedule, you should find a rhythm that feels right for you. The appeal is in being able to change and try new things, making sure the approach you select fits in perfectly with your way of living.

Creating a customized fasting schedule becomes a major theme for you on your journey. Setting realistic goals begins with evaluating your current state of health and fitness. The focus lies in developing a routine that is not only efficient but also long-lasting. Staying on track and reaping the complete benefits of intermittent fasting is ensured by tracking your progress and making any modifications along the way.

Meal preparation and nutrition are important themes in this story. Your daily routine should incorporate maintaining a balance of macronutrients, emphasizing nutrient-dense foods, and researching hydration and supplementation techniques. Not only should you refrain from eating, but you should also feed your body with satisfying and tasty meals that support your fasting way of life.

There is a toolbox of ways to help with the difficulty of controlling appetite and cravings. It then becomes a matter of knowing your body's cues and acting accordingly to overcome hunger. In order to address cravings and create a long-lasting, positive relationship with food, it is important to address both psychological and physical factors.

Exercise adds a new level of complexity to your intermittent fasting journey, but it also has enormous benefits. The benefits to your general well-being are increased when workouts are customized to your age and fitness level and take into account the mutually beneficial interaction between exercise and fasting.

But it's important to carefully consider any potential health risks and safety measures. Intermittent fasting is a safe and useful tool in your health toolkit as long as you consult medical professionals, take care of any pre-existing illnesses, and stay attentive to your well-being.

We honor the accomplishments and motivational tales of women over 50 who have adopted intermittent fasting as we draw this story to a close. Their personal stories provide a source of inspiration, demonstrating the resiliency, tenacity, and happiness that come with this way of living.

For women over 50, intermittent fasting is essentially a dynamic and individualized approach to well-being rather than merely a regimen. It's about tuning into your body's rhythm, personalizing your path, and relishing the rich mosaic of encounters encountered along the way. With every step you take toward a healthier, more vibrant you, may this summary be as a gentle reminder that your road to improved health is uniquely yours.

Encouragement and Motivation

It's admirable that a woman over 50 has decided to start intermittent fasting; it shows how dedicated you are to your health and wellbeing. When you embark on this lifestyle shift, it's important to keep in mind that your mental toughness and optimistic outlook will be your greatest assets, independent of any physical changes.

Let me start by congratulating yourself for making this decision. Recognize that although change can be difficult, it frequently serves as the impetus for amazing development and transformation. There is a thriving community of women who embrace intermittent fasting, each with their own narrative, problems, and victories, so you are not alone on this path. Although your path is exclusively yours, it is also shared with many like-minded people, and you are a part of a strong support system.

Be kind to yourself as you learn to live with the rhythms of intermittent fasting. Results may not come right away, so patience is essential. Savor the little triumphs along the way: the days you easily follow your fasting schedule, the times you choose your food carefully, and the moments you experience an energy boost. All of these indicate that the adjustments you're making are having a favorable effect on your body.

It's critical to see intermittent fasting as an empowered lifestyle rather than a restrictive diet. Accept the flexibility it offers and choose when to eat instead of what to avoid. This method promotes a better connection with eating while letting you enjoy the things you enjoy. Recall that the goal is to fuel your body in a manner that promotes your general wellbeing, not to starve it.

There will be times when the path seems difficult and your dedication falters. Think back on the more profound motivations for your choice to experiment with intermittent fasting at these times. Reconnect with your motivations, whether they are related to bettering your health, increasing your energy, or just feeling more self-assured. When things get tough, use your image of the woman you want to be to help you get through it.

Embrace a supportive network of friends, family, and/or online groups as your immediate surroundings. Talk about your experiences, give advice, and get ideas from those who have been down a similar road. When you most need it, the combined experience of individuals who have successfully negotiated the challenges of intermittent fasting can offer insightful advice and support.

Observe the mental and emotional changes that are taking place inside of you in addition to the physical ones. The goal of intermittent fasting is to develop a mindset that promotes acceptance and love for oneself, not only to change the way your body looks. Accept the increased mental clarity and focus that come with fasting. Your eating habits won't be the only areas of your life that will benefit from this mental toughness.

Recall that your body is an amazing machine that can heal and adapt. Have faith in the process and give your body time to become used to the new rhythm. Pay attention to its cues and be kind in your response. If things don't go as planned or you have setbacks, view them as teaching moments rather than failures. Your journey of intermittent fasting is dynamic, just like life itself.

Honor the distinctiveness of your encounter. It's acceptable if your journey will not look like everyone else's. Savor the little adjustments and the sense of independence that come with managing your health. Recognize the strength of your fortitude and the bravery required to welcome change.

Remind yourself that you are able to accomplish amazing things when you are feeling doubtful. Intermittent fasting is a journey of self-discovery, a celebration of the amazing woman you are becoming, and a monument to your power. Carry the torch of inspiration and guidance along this route, lighting the way for those who might choose to walk in your footsteps.

It is important to embrace the process, celebrate your accomplishments, and remember that intermittent fasting is not just about changing your physical appearance but also about developing your inner strength, confidence, and inspiration as a woman. This is something you can handle!

Recipe Ideas

○ **RECIPE 1**

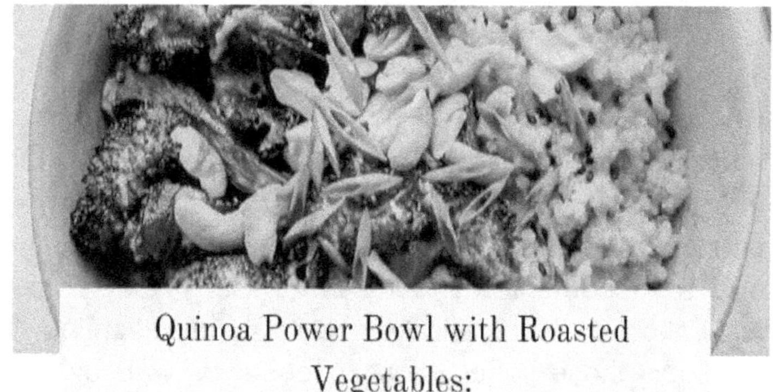

Quinoa Power Bowl with Roasted Vegetables:

PREPPING TIME: 15 MIN   COOKING TIME: 30 MIN

Ingredients

- medium sweet potato, peeled and cut into 1-inch cubes
- 1 medium beet, trimmed, peeled and cut into 1-inch cubes
- 2 cups broccoli florets
- Extra-virgin olive oil
- Salt
- Black pepper
- 4 cups mixed greens
- 1 cup cooked quinoa
- 1/4 cup almonds
- 1 tablespoon fresh cilantro

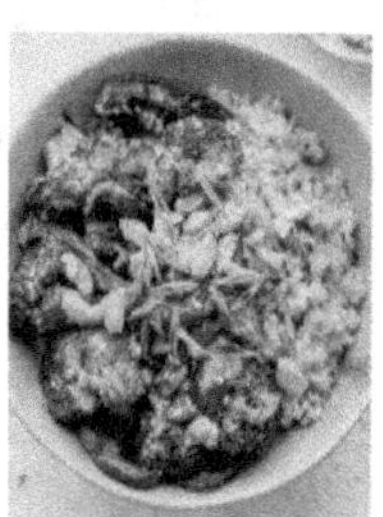

Direction

- Set the oven's temperature to 400 degrees.

- Combine the diced sweet potatoes, roughly 2 tsp olive oil, and a dash of salt and pepper in a medium-sized bowl. Transfer them to a large baking sheet with a rim. To prevent the beets' color from transferring onto the sweet potatoes, repeat this process with the cubed beets and place them on the same rimmed baking sheet next to them. Place the baking sheet in the oven that has been preheated, and roast for ten to twelve minutes.

- Toss the broccoli florets in the same bowl with a sprinkling of salt and pepper and roughly 2 tsp. olive oil. Take out of the oven the baking sheet and place the broccoli florets next to the beets. After that, put the baking sheet back in the oven and roast everything for a further ten to twelve minutes. After removing, place aside to cool to ambient temperature.

- In the meantime, whisk together all of the dressing's components in a small bowl until well combined. You can thin the dressing with a tablespoon of water if it's too thick—this will depend on the brand of tahini paste you use.

- Divide the cooked quinoa and greens equally between two bowls to assemble the bowls. Add the roasted veggies, almonds, and cilantro on top. Pour in the dressing. Serve right away.

Picture a colorful bowl filled with nutty quinoa, perfectly roasted vegetables, and a drizzle of olive oil. This power-packed dish is rich in essential nutrients, providing a hearty and satisfying meal during your eating window.

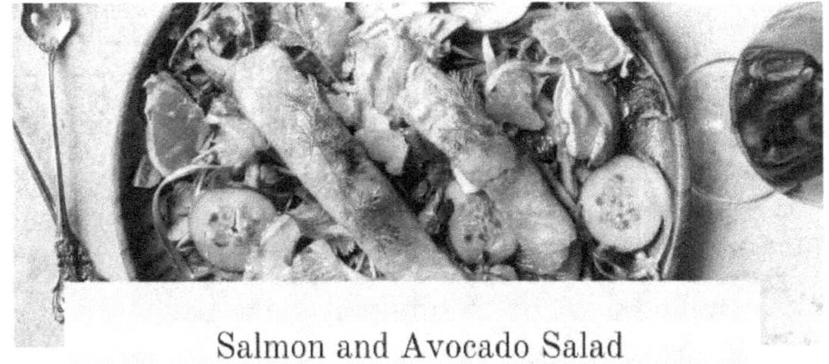

Salmon and Avocado Salad

PREPPING TIME: 15 MIN   COOKING TIME: 30 MIN

Ingredients

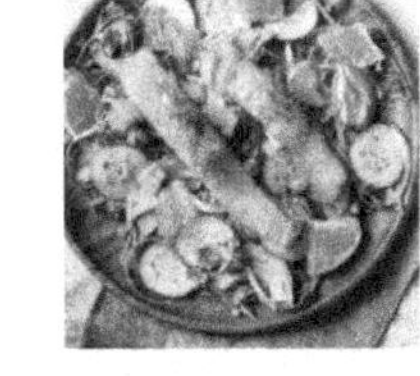

- ½ cup loosely packed fresh dill, plus more for garnish
- 2 tablespoons water
- 2 tablespoons lemon juice
- 2 tablespoons white-wine vinegar
- 1 teaspoon Dijon mustard
- 1 small clove garlic
- 2 avocados, chopped, divided
- ¼ cup extra-virgin olive oil, plus 1 teaspoon, divided
- ½ teaspoon salt, divided
- 4 (5 ounce) skinless salmon fillets
- ¼ teaspoon ground pepper
- 3 cups spring mix salad greens
- 2 cups thinly sliced red cabbage
- 1 cup matchstick carrots

Direction

- In a blender, place the dill, water, vinegar, lemon juice, mustard, garlic, 1/2 cup avocado, 1/4 cup oil, and 1/4 teaspoon salt. Process for 30 seconds or until smooth. Store in the fridge until needed.

- In a large cast-iron skillet, heat the remaining 1 teaspoon oil over medium-high heat. Evenly sprinkle the fish with the remaining 1/4 teaspoon salt and pepper. Place the salmon in the pan and cook for about 4 minutes, or until it becomes golden on the bottom and is mostly opaque around the edges. After carefully turning the filets, turn off the heat. Give the filets two to three minutes to cook thoroughly in the pan.

- In a large bowl, combine salad greens, cabbage, carrots, and the leftover dressing; toss gently to coat evenly. Arrange the salad onto four dishes and sprinkle the leftover avocado on top. Place a salmon filet on top of each salad and, if wanted, add more dill as a garnish.

Make a light salad by combining the healthy omega-3 benefits of salmon with creamy avocados. Along with being heart-healthy, the combination is a delicious blend of flavors and sensations. To add a little kick, drizzle with a little vinaigrette.

○ **RECIPE 3**

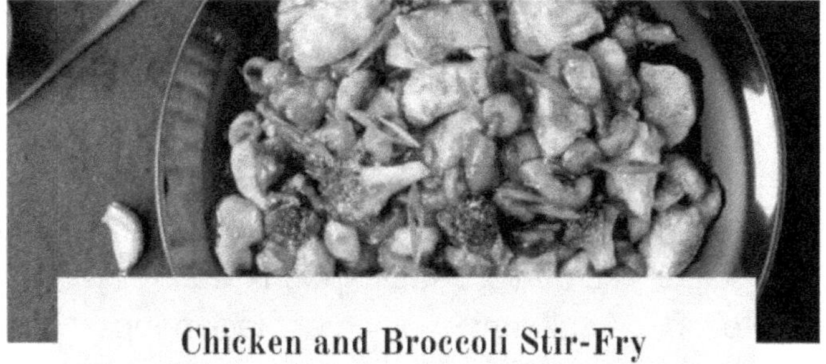

Chicken and Broccoli Stir-Fry

PREPPING TIME: 15 MIN   COOKING TIME: 30 MIN

Ingredients

- Chicken breast (about 2 breasts), cubed
- 3 scallions, whites only, thinly sliced on a bias
- 2 tablespoons sugar
- 1 tablespoon dark sesame oil
- 1 tablespoon dry sherry
- 1 tablespoon soy sauce
- 2 cloves garlic, minced
- 1-inch piece peeled fresh ginger, minced
- 1 tablespoon, plus 1 teaspoon cornstarch
- Kosher salt and freshly ground black pepper
- About 1/3 cup water
- 3 tablespoons vegetable oil
- 5 to 6 cups broccoli florets and sliced stalks (keep the 2 cuts separate)
- 3/4 to 1 teaspoon red chili flakes, optional
- 1 tablespoon hoisin sauce
- Ttoasted sesame seeds, for serving, optional
- Jasmine rice, for serving, optional

<u>Direction</u>

- Combine the chicken with the scallion whites, sugar, sesame oil, sherry, soy sauce, half of the ginger and garlic, one teaspoon cornstarch, and one teaspoon salt in a medium-sized bowl. Let marinate for fifteen minutes at room temperature. In a small bowl, whisk together the remaining 1 tablespoon cornstarch and 1/3 cup water. Set aside.

- A big nonstick skillet should be heated to high heat. Heat after adding 1 tablespoon of vegetable oil. Stir-fry the broccoli stems for 30 seconds after adding them. Stir in the remaining ginger and garlic, 2 tablespoons water, 1/4 teaspoon salt, and a pinch of black pepper. Add the florets as well. Stir-fry for about 2 minutes, or until the broccoli is brilliant green but still crunchy. Move to a platter.

- Reheat the skillet to a high temperature before adding the final two teaspoons of vegetable oil. If using, mix in the chicken and red pepper flakes. Stir-fry for 3 minutes or until the chicken starts to become a light brown and loses its raw hue. When the broccoli is back in the skillet, add the hoisin sauce and mix to fully reheat. To thicken, add the cornstarch mixture that was set aside and bring it to a boil. If more water is required to thin the sauce, add it. If desired, add salt and pepper after tasting.

- Mound the stir-fry on a serving platter or divide among 4 plates and garnish with sesame seeds; serve with rice.

Stir-frying some chicken and broccoli will quickly and flavorfully elevate your dinner. Choose a stir-fry sauce with lots of flavor, crisp broccoli florets, and lean chicken breast. Serve over cauliflower rice for a filling and well-rounded dinner.

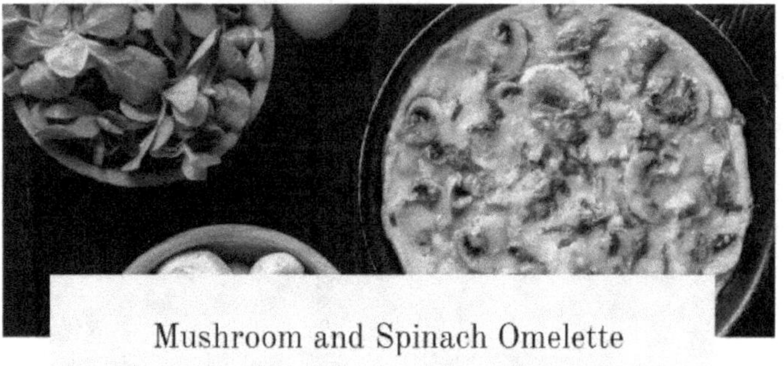

Mushroom and Spinach Omelette

PREPPING TIME: 10 MIN   COOKING TIME: 25 MIN

Ingredients

- ½4 egg
- 1/2 cup chopped spinach
- 1/2 cup chopped mushroom
- 1 tablespoon parmesan cheese
- 1 tablespoon cheese-cheddar
- 2 teaspoon garlic powder
- Black pepper as required
- Chilli flakes as required
- 1/2 cup chopped onion
- 2 tablespoon virgin olive oil

salt as required

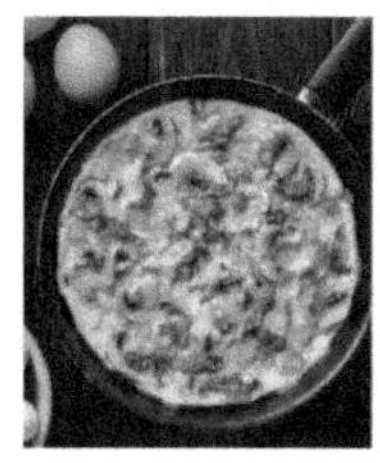

<u>Direction</u>

- In a large bowl, combine the eggs, parmesan, cheddar, black pepper, salt, garlic powder, and red chili flakes. Whisk well to achieve a creamy texture. This is how to make an incredible egg recipe.

- After the oil is hot enough, place a pan over medium heat and add some olive oil. Add the

chopped mushrooms and onions, and heat until
they start to brown slightly.

- Add chopped spinach and let it cook for 5
  minutes on medium heat. Keep stirring
  occasionally. Evenly pour the egg mixture in the
  pan and spread it over the tossed veggies.

- Cook the egg until it's done. Flip the omelet over
  and reheat it. Toast is served hot!

- The omelet will taste better if the egg white and
  yolk are whisked separately and beaten until
  foamy, giving the omelet a fluffy texture.

A high-protein omelet loaded with fresh spinach and
sautéed mushrooms is a great way to start the day. This
breakfast alternative keeps you feeling full and
energized throughout the morning, plus it's really simple
to prepare.

○ **RECIPE 5**

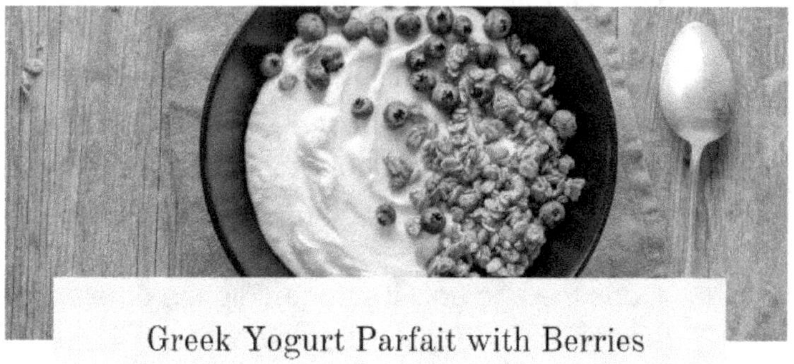

Greek Yogurt Parfait with Berries

PREPPING TIME: 10 MIN   COOKING TIME: 25 MIN

Ingredients

- 1 cup fresh strawberries sliced
- ¼ cup granulated sugar
- 1 cup vanilla Greek yogurt
- ½ cup fresh blueberries
- ½ cup granola

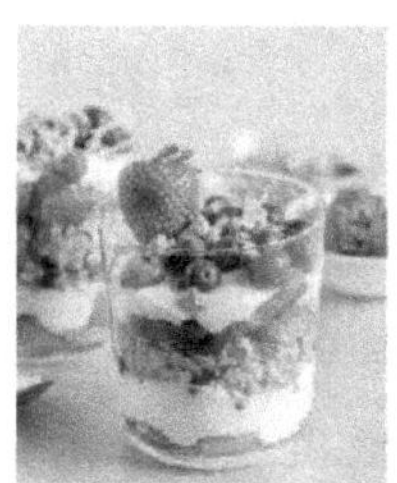

Direction

- In a bowl, combine the strawberries and sugar; whisk to mix. Refrigerate for half an hour or overnight with a cover on.
- Split half of the strawberries between two transparent glasses.
- Top with half of the Greek yogurt.
- Top with half of the blueberries.
- Top with all of the granola.

- Continue by adding another layer of blueberries, another layer of Greek yogurt, and another layer of strawberries. (granola, red, white, blue, red, white, blue)
- For optimal consistency, serve right away.

Sooth your sweet tooth with a parfait made of Greek yogurt. Greek yogurt can be layered with fresh berries and a dash of almonds to make a delicious snack or dessert. This alternative offers a dosage of probiotics for intestinal health in addition to being delicious.

14-Day Meal Plan

	Break-Fast (12:00 PM)	**Lunch (3:00 PM)**	**Dinner (7:00 PM)**
DAY 1	Greek Yogurt Parfait with Berries and Nuts	Grilled Chicken Salad with Mixed Greens and Avocado	Baked Salmon with Quinoa and Steamed Broccoli
DAY 2	Scrambled Eggs with Spinach and Tomatoes	Chickpea and Vegetable Stir-Fry	Turkey Meatballs with Zucchini Noodles
DAY 3	Smoothie with Spinach, Banana, and Almond Milk	Lentil Soup with a Side of Mixed Greens	Grilled Shrimp with Brown Rice and Asparagus

DAY 4	Oatmeal with Chia Seeds and Fresh Berries	Quinoa Salad with Roasted Vegetables and Feta Cheese	Baked Chicken Breast with Sweet Potato and Green Beans
DAY 5	Cottage Cheese with Pineapple and Almonds	Spinach and Feta Stuffed Chicken Breast	Stir-Fried Tofu with Brown Rice and Broccoli
DAY 6	Whole Grain Toast with Smashed Avocado and Poached Eggs	Quinoa Bowl with Black Beans, Corn, and Salsa	Grilled Mahi-Mahi with Quinoa and Roasted Brussels Sprouts
DAY 7	Greek Yogurt Parfait with Berries and Nuts	Grilled Chicken Salad with Mixed Greens and Avocado	Baked Salmon with Quinoa and Steamed Broccoli

DAY 8	Scrambled Eggs with Spinach and Tomatoes	Chickpea and Vegetable Stir-Fry	Turkey Meatballs with Zucchini Noodles
DAY 9	Smoothie with Spinach, Banana, and Almond Milk	Lentil Soup with a Side of Mixed Greens	Grilled Shrimp with Brown Rice and Asparagus
DAY 10	Oatmeal with Chia Seeds and Fresh Berries	Quinoa Salad with Roasted Vegetables and Feta Cheese	Baked Chicken Breast with Sweet Potato and Green Beans
DAY 11	Cottage Cheese with Pineapple and Almonds	Spinach and Feta Stuffed Chicken Breast	Stir-Fried Tofu with Brown Rice and Broccoli
DAY 12	Whole Grain Toast with Smashed Avocado and	Quinoa Bowl with Black Beans, Corn, and Salsa	Grilled Mahi-Mahi with Quinoa and Roasted Brussels

	Poached Eggs		Sprouts
DAY 13	Greek Yogurt Parfait with Berries and Nuts	Grilled Chicken Salad with Mixed Greens and Avocado	Baked Salmon with Quinoa and Steamed Broccoli

DAY 14	Chia Seed Pudding with Sliced Mango	Turkey and Vegetable Wrap with Whole Grain Tortilla	Grilled Salmon with Quinoa Salad and Steamed Asparagus

www.ingramcontent.com/pod-product-compliance
Lightning Source LLC
Chambersburg PA
CBHW070846260726
48661CB00004B/1266